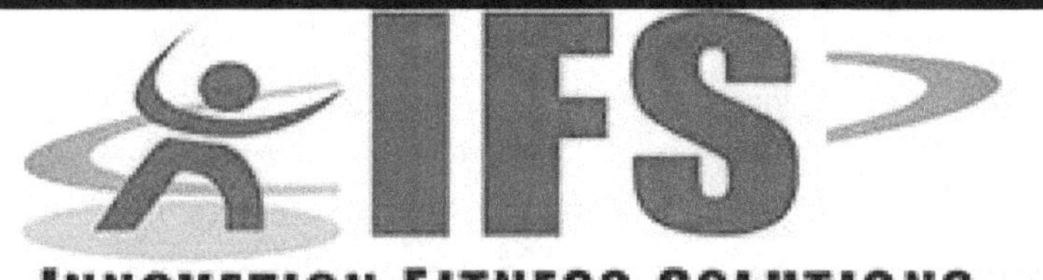

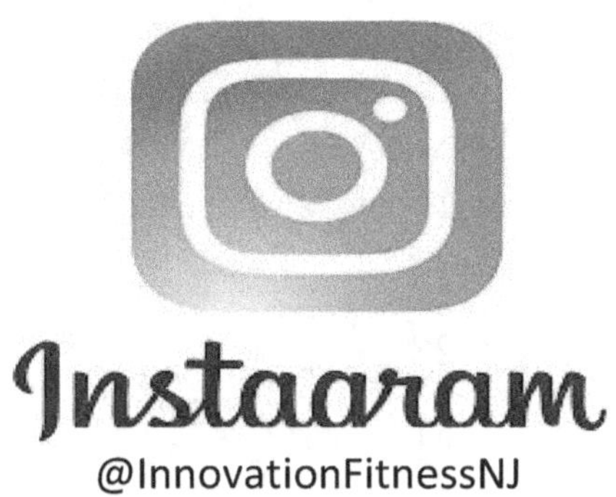

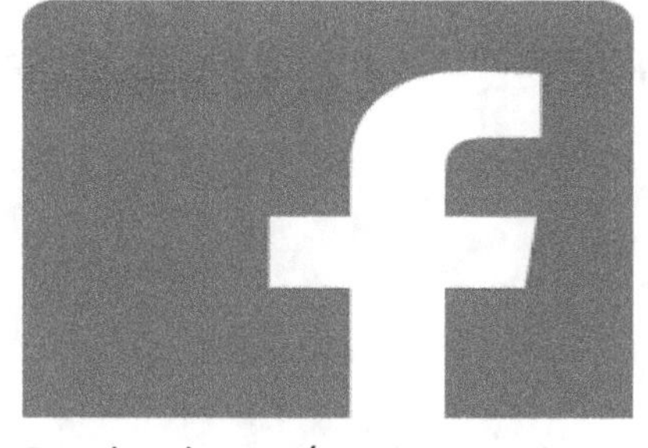

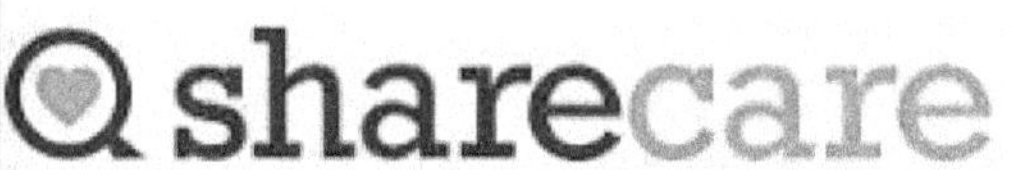

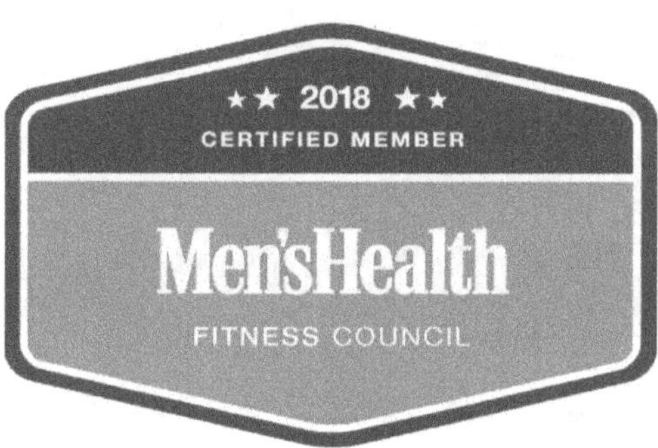

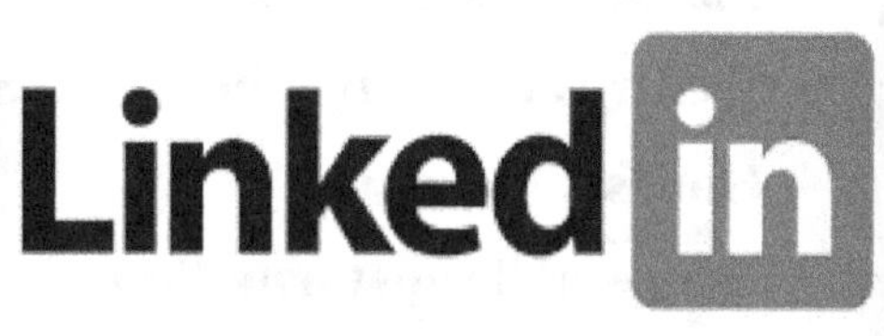

Written by: Robert J DeVito, BS

Edited by: Kelsey Pezzuti, BS, MS, CISSN

Edited and Designed by: Lindsey Wormald, BA

This book is not intended as a substitute for the medical advice of Physicians or Dieticians. The reader should regularly consult a physician in matters relating to his/her health and particularly with respect to any symptoms that may require diagnosis or medical attention.

ISBN-13:
978-1985789463

ISBN-10:
1985789469

Copyright 2018

Robert J DeVito founded Innovation Fitness Solutions, LLC in 2000. Innovation Fitness began as a health club consulting company, providing business management, staff education and fitness program systems for commercial health clubs to provide results for the gym-goer.

In 2006, we changed direction by relieving the gym of staffing and programming issues. IFS brought a complete "done for you" system into our franchised gyms. After some more success and even more frustration, in 2008, we eliminated the middleman entirely and opened our first Wellness and Weight Loss facility in the Northern New Jersey area. Our programming and coaching options account for the Physical – Mental – Emotional – Environmental strategies required for long-term success. We offer a WHOLEistic approach to life. Complete, solution-based programming delivered by caring experts to improve Health, Wellness and Weight Loss.

Commitment + Support + Education + Motivation = Results for Life.

CORE VALUES

INNOVATION

The drive to succeed is shared by our entire team. We are
passionate about helping our clients live better lives. We strive to
deliver solutions based on effective long-term programming.
By recognizing our clients wants and needs and refusing to
IFS leads the way in creating and producing outstanding
accept shortcuts we remain at the pinnacle of the fitness industry.
programming delivered by our highly skilled and caring team.

INTEGRITY

No company can successfully survive without integrity.
Our communication is simple and honest. We maintain strict
standards for education, communication and work relentlessly
towards creating a positive, respectful and supportive
environment, Excellence and Teamwork are two attributes that
should be expected of our team.

IMPACT

IFS provides our clients with unparalleled service, programs and
training. Our solutions impact the lives of our clients and their
families lives by providing real-life results that are "WHOLEistic",
progressive and sustainable.

RESULTS FOR LIFE

f /innovationfitness   www.innovationfitness.net

Performance Coaching

Welcome to Innovation Fitness Solutions. Everyone on our team is excited to help you achieve your goals and aid you in your transformation. We have had the honor of helping thousands of people succeed in their fitness quest. IFS is your last step in achieving the goals and dreams you set for yourself. We do not promise magic diets, amazing results without effort or magical pills and potions. We are specialists in Coaching. We consider the physical, mental, environmental and emotional needs for you to be successful long term. With our guidance and support and with your determination and persistence you will achieve remarkable results. <u>That is our promise.</u>

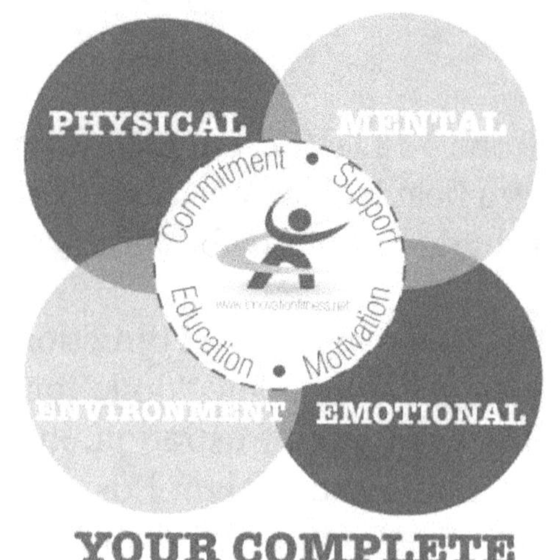

A Program Overview and Philosophy:

The stated goal for most of us is to "lose weight"; however, when we break down our desires and gain all the facts of what our goals entail – we determine that we want much more than "just" weight loss. Our goal becomes TRANSFORMATION - to change the shape of our bodies by reducing body fat, maintaining muscle tissue, increasing our energy levels, and improving our overall health. Our "Big Picture" goals are centered on finding balance, peace and happiness and improving all the facets of our wellness. ***Weight loss is a <u>side-effect</u> of better habits;*** not choosing the "diet of the week" or the magical series of exercises. It is a cumulative effect of coaching yourself to create a different and better, more consistent YOU. ***Simply stated, to lose body weight, calories expended must be greater than calories consumed.*** This simple equation is the First Law of Thermodynamics. It is inarguable and remains true. However, it is one small component of what you need to do for the transformation that you desire. Basically, it is more than JUST calorie intake and expenditure that counts. The focus of the **IFS Weight Management System** is to help you change your body composition and improve your overall health through controlling energy while increasing **<u>vitality</u>**. Weight Loss and Health Goals are not separate entities. They are dramatically intertwined with every choice affecting everything else. Maintaining a focus on what is necessary to bring you continual progress.

The **IFS System** is a scientifically based weight management and wellness system created to provide safe and effective results to help you look and feel better. It is designed to work with your eating habits and current lifestyle. We will provide you with the knowledge necessary to help modify your lifestyle in a step-by-step approach that will allow you to attain and maintain your results.

WHAT DO YOU TRULY WANT IN LIFE?   WHY?

The **first step** in creating your M.A.P. (My Action Plan) is to choose a PRIMARY Goal.

FAT LOSS

Who's it for?
Individuals interested in transforming their physiques through a proven, long-term solution. Transformation from the inside out.

What to expect...
The ultimate coaching experience
Mindset training (see "dieting" differently)
Insights into your helping/hurting habits
Proper goal setting
Become consistent and accountable
Remain positive
Overcome weight loss plateaus
Find your eating style
Balance hormones
Provide nutritional support
Create/maintain an energy deficit
Increase strength and energy
Appropriate and safe fitness plan
Maximize energy expenditure

HEALTH & WELLNESS

Who's it for?
Individuals interested in reaching their highest level of health, while gaining improved, overall wellness.

What to expect...
Focus - Achieving optimal health and wellness is a journey of discovery.
Mindfulness training
Relaxation techniques
Stress reduction
Improve patience and remain present
Food education
Always choose your best foods
Eating for health and longevity
Nutritional support products
Improve fitness
Improve cardiovascular fitness
Enhance daily activities
Prehab (strengthen back and core)

FITNESS & PERFORMANCE

Who's it for?
Individuals looking to gain muscle, increase strength and improve athletic performance.

What to expect...
Focus - Achieving maximum growth and performance requires strategies that challenge the body at a very high level, but also create an environment for proper recovery.
Performance increases
Increase mental awareness
Maximize workout intensity
Proper training cycles
Recovery
Sleep patterns
Flexibility and mobility work
Stress relief techniques
Performance nutrition
Meal composition/timing
Advanced nutritional support products

STEP TWO - The coaches will assign you a Skill Level so together, we can choose the appropriate Group Training Sessions for you to begin with based on your goals and needs.

LEVEL 1	RECRUIT	I AM NEW TO ALL OF THIS
LEVEL 2	CONTENDER	I AM STARTING TO FEEL STRONG
LEVEL 3	VETERAN	I HAVE BEEN DOING FITNESS FOR A WHILE
LEVEL 4	ALL STAR	I AM IN GOOD SHAPE
LEVEL 5	HALL OF FAMER	I AM AN ACHIEVER AMONG MORTALS

The **third step** is to determine which sessions you should attend based on your needs.

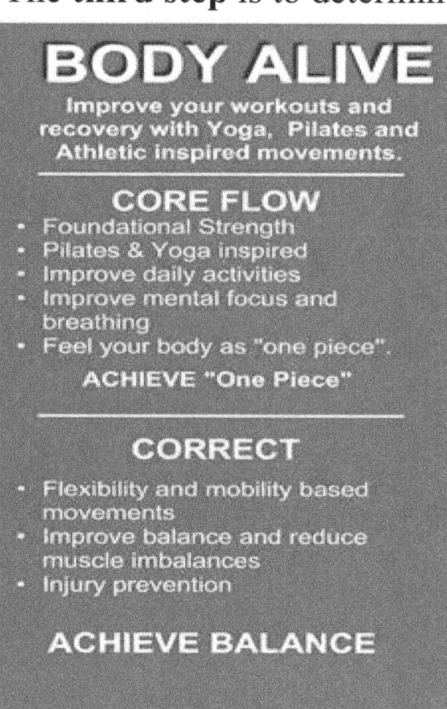

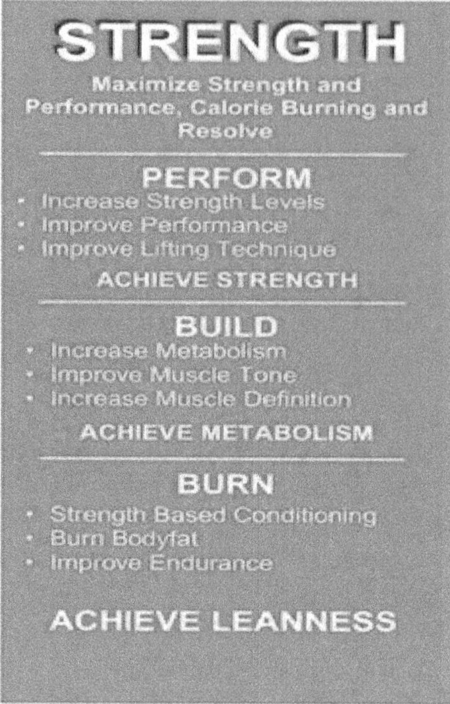

As you progress in skill, conditioning and confidence, your sessions will need to be adjusted to continue progress.

Typically, we suggest 4 weekly sessions: 2 - Strength Sessions, 1 - Body Alive Session and 1 - Coaching session. For experienced exercisers, you should consider 3 Strength sessions, 1- Body Alive session and 1 – Coaching session weekly.

Discussing your specific goals and needs with your Coach will help us direct you during your evolution. As your skill and fitness levels improve, your session selection may need to change.

Finally, to avoid adapting to the stimulus and to continue progress in strength and fat burning, we use a periodization model for our Group Training sessions. This model allows us to focus on specific tasks and outcomes for a desired amount of time, then switching to a different focus. Not only does this prevent stagnation in your body, it provides recuperation too and something to look forward to in your training.

Example – one month your Strength Sessions will be focused on building metabolism and strength, the next month would see the focus switch to maximizing body fat loss. In an ideal world, we would be able to accomplish these things in a constant, linear fashion, but, unfortunately our body's physiology does not work that way. To simplify this a bit, we have provided information on the distinct types of training sessions we use and information on "other" popular modalities.

4 Diverse Types of Workouts:
Weight-based, Cardio-based, Mixed & Fun/Fitness.

When you view exercise through the lens of body-change, and sustainable results, these four methods reveal a path to long-term change. For body transformation, these methods are not interchangeable and certainly, are not equal. The priority for body transformation should always be strength-based workouts with conditioning added in periodically and planned. Most people believe that all workouts and diets lead to the same results. This is a mistaken thought process, just like studying Spanish will not teach you to speak French, fitness is finite and specific. The correct programming yields results. The incorrect program creates effort without results.

1. **Weight Based. Strength BUILD** – Weightlifting to build metabolism and increase "toning". You know you are doing this type of workout when you are gritting your teeth, and basically feel your entire body shutter under the weight. For the best results during Strength – Build and Strength – Perform, you should choose loads that only allow for 6-12 repetitions. If you are not feeling the load within 10 reps, you will need to increase your effort to experience strength gains and body change.
- Examples – Squatting, Deadlifting, lifting overhead, heavy sled work, Straight or Supersets.
- Benefits – Increase in strength. Increase in metabolism (ability to burn calories). Strength training is the only way to build muscle, which burns calories and increases "tone".

2. **BURN/Conditioning.** These types of workouts are faster paced, with short rest periods. Generally, they are performed with lighter weights and higher repetition strength work. The focus is not on lifting heavy things, it is on maximizing calorie burn DURING the session. You may feel some light exertion in your muscles, but, mainly, these sessions are felt in the lungs.
- Examples – Jump rope, Sled work, Burpees, Kettlebell Complexes
- Benefits – Once Strength - Build has added muscle, you can use it to maximize fat loss for 3- 4-week intervals.

3. **PERFORM** – sessions combining moderate lifts and conditioning. We also introduce new movements during PERFORM sessions. We focus on form improvement and new skill acquisition to add to your exercise arsenal safely and effectively.

4. **Fun/Fitness** – This is any activity that is not listed above. These activities may or may not directly affect body composition.
- Examples – Walking, hiking, Zumba class, Bootcamps, Pilates, Yoga, endless cardio. Basically, all these activities fall under the category of "Accessory Work".

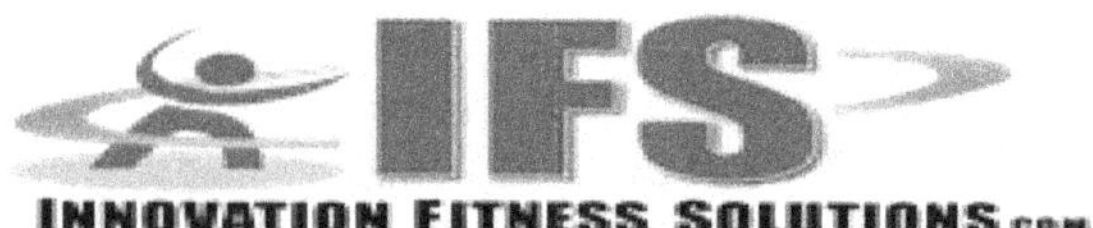

Choosing Your Training Sessions
The diverse types of Personal Training

Private Training - One trainer to one client. Private training is best suited long-term for people with special needs such as athletes or individuals with prior injuries, or, realistically, more introverted people that do not wish to be in a group. For most people, 1-2 months of Private training should be enough to prepare them to move on to the next level of training.

- Special Consideration – We like for members to schedule at least one Private Training Session per month as a check-in, to refine movements, learn new movements and get individual guidance towards their goals.

Partner Training – Session performed with one trainer and two clients. Ideally, both clients would be of similar personality and skill level. A trainer can devise a plan for everyone to attain their goals while providing a good amount of attention to each client. A few benefits to Partner training are reduced cost, camaraderie, connectedness, and motivation. There is also an additional layer of accountability as you are much more likely to attend sessions when you know that someone else is expecting you and counting on you.

Small Group Training – Sessions with one trainer and 3-4 clients. Small Group Training (SGT) is an excellent choice for many people with fitness and weight loss goals. This environment allows for a good amount of individualization and is incredibly motivating. SGT benefits far outweigh anything lost from Private or Partner training. SGT is fun and intense and is a cost-effective choice as a long-term, results-driven training option. You are sure to work harder in this arena and create lasting relationships while being provided specialized attention.

Large Group Training – Sessions with 1-2 trainers and 8-15 clients. This type of training is primarily for intermediate to advanced exercisers, not a beginner or novice. This environment is generally incredibly motivating and fun. It is highly cost-effective and is a great option for long-term training. Meshing SGT and LGT sessions is great for most clients, so we always can address specific goals and needs that you can execute in the larger group sessions. This class style has become increasingly popular over the past few years for several reasons:

- Multiple studies show that people exercise harder and for longer in groups.
- The style of class has a lower cost of entry than other Personal or Group Training programs.
- Classes are intense and challenging.
- People learn to be more creative in their own personal workouts.

How do I get started?

We begin each client with **PRIVATE** (one client to one trainer) sessions for a 1-2-month period. This allows us to be confident that the client is prepared for success in their next level of training. We build a base level of conditioning, allow the client the time to learn proper movement patterns, gain confidence in their understanding of performance and mentally and physically ready to succeed in a group. Where you go next should be decided on between you and your coach.

Choosing the appropriate GROUP Training Sessions
An individual desiring FAT LOSS as their primary goal should attend -
- STRENGTH TRAINING sessions, 3 days per week.
- Recovery and rejuvenation sessions (Body Alive) at least 1 day per week.
- Increase their education (Coaching) to help achieve their goals in a simplified way at least one day per week.

An individual desiring Health & Wellness as their primary goal should attend -
- STRENGTH TRAINING sessions, 2 days per week.
- Recovery and rejuvenation sessions (Body Alive) at least 2 days per week.
- Increase their education (Coaching) to help achieve their goals in a simplified way at least one day per week.

An individual desiring Fitness & Performance as their primary goal should attend -
- STRENGTH TRAINING sessions, 3 - 4 days per week.
- Recovery and rejuvenation sessions (Body Alive) at least 1 day per week.
- Increase their education (Coaching) to help achieve their goals in a simplified way at least one day per week.

By following our tried and proven system, you are sure to remain safe, motivated and progressing quickly towards your goals.

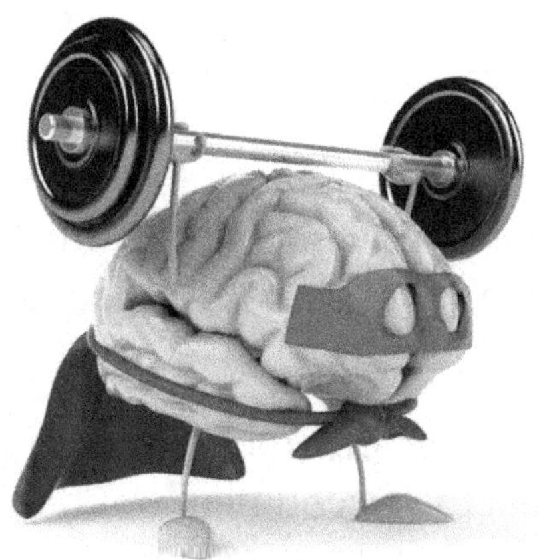

Maximizing your Membership Experience

<u>**Your integrity**</u> - The training client's code of responsibility:

I take **total responsibility** for my health and my results (Food, Fitness, and Focus). I understand that everyone faces challenges, which I will treat as obstacles that might take me on a different fitness path; I will not treat them as barriers that will prevent me from reaching my goals. I understand true health and wellness is about the continued journey, not only about reaching a short-term goal. I understand my current physical condition is my fault and no one else's, and only I have the power to change myself. I acknowledge that with proper coaching and by remaining coachable I will be much more likely to have my ultimate success. I also understand my health, physical condition and wellness is the most valuable thing I own and that I must invest in myself regularly to live my life at a higher level of well-being. I will commit to do the work necessary to make changes and I understand that what I put into this endeavor is what I will get out of it.

1. I will find a coach whom I trust and stick to the plan. I will not try and outthink my trained professional.

2. I will accept who I am now and not try to be the person I was physically 20 years ago.

3. I understand that no matter how many times a week I go to the gym, there is no magic workout that will overcome a poor lifestyle. If I want substantial change, I must make change, in not only how I approach fitness, but how I live too.

4. I will always remember that there will be days when I just don't feel like it and even the act of showing up and getting it done is far superior to doing nothing at all.

5. Good coaches lead but aren't magicians. I still must do the work if I want the change. My fitness is my responsibility.

6. I understand that the goal of any fitness plan is the quality of life. Looking good is nice but living healthy and feeling great is everything in life and fitness.

7. I realize that about 99% of all the crap on Facebook and Instagram may not be true and I will trust my coach instead of the magic exercise or supplement of the week.

8. I will not lie to my coach about food, or wine, or what I ate Sunday watching the game. And no matter what I say, I realize my body can't lie and what I ate is what I wore in today, so I might as well as write it all down.

9. My goal is to get to the point where I understand that fitness is motion, and motion is life, and the best day of my life is when I just go out for a long walk for the simple pleasure of moving that day.

10. I will understand that my coach is a professional, the same as everyone else who supports me in life, such as my doctor, accountant or chiropractor, and that I understand he or she needs to get paid decent money for putting up with my nonsense every week.

Finally, as a client, I swear to come in everyday in a good mood, not be bitchy or arrogant. I will be polite to the other members, respect the gym and my coach and most importantly, I swear to just do the work with a smile and a thank you for a good workout.

Improving your performance and enjoyment during Training Sessions

1. **Prepare** - Attend your sessions mentally prepared. Come in to work hard and in your best mood possible. Be prepared to leave in an even better mood.
   - Eat a snack or meal 60 – 90 minutes prior to a training session and be sure to drink water before and during exercise.
   - Take care of your basic needs like taking a Multi-Vitamin, ensuring adequate rest and recovery, thinking positively and reaching out for support when needed.
   - Arrive 10-15 minutes early for the sessions to warm-up by using the cardiovascular equipment and to perform light flexibility exercises.

2. **Coaching** - If your goal is Fat Loss, be sure to attend the weekly group lifestyle coaching sessions. This session will increase the likelihood of your success by helping you prepare and plan for the other 23 hours of the day.

3. **Communicate** – Having an open dialogue with your Coaches and fellow members is imperative to you getting what you need to be successful. Informing your Coach if you are struggling during a workout, having a tough day, have a new pain or need a modification are all important aspects of ensuring your safety, helping to create a fantastic experience every time you are here and maximizing your time. Not communicating simply makes our job (and yours) to help more difficult and your experience gets lessened.
   - Monitor your wellbeing during Fitness Sessions, communicating with the Coach if you feel faint, overly fatigued, dizzy and/or nauseous.
   - Work up to your current skill level and physical ability. Be intelligent about your exertion and push yourself, but do not put yourself into a position of potential injury.

4. **Respect the equipment -** Please do your best to not drop, slam or abuse the equipment. Part of keeping our costs down is maintaining the integrity of the equipment. Think of the equipment as community goods. If you damage them, you damage them for everyone.

5. **Rest -** There is no need to work out 7 days per week. Take rest days that are rest days. Recovery is an imperative part of a fitness lifestyle. If you do not recover from training, you create difficulty in attaining your goals. You will not be able to maximize your performance during workouts due to this lack of recovery and hence, your results will suffer.

6. **Don't let life get in the way** - On the flip side, don't take too many rest days. We don't want to get into the habit of making attending your sessions an intermittent occurrence.

One or two days on followed by five or six days off will interrupt the workout routine you've worked hard to establish.

7. **Make as many modifications as necessary -** Contrary to widespread belief, your goal is not to perform every workout to the maximum intensity possible. Your coach programs your workouts for you to feel a stimulus, at a planned capacity, for a specified amount of time. Modify your workout to meet this intention, not your ego. Each workout is a part of a program, with intention and desired outcomes for a goal, not a standalone event.

8. **Do your best -** Give your best effort every single day. You will feel like you can take on the world some days, and others, not so much. The days that you do not feel like exercising, it is important to show up and do what you can. That effort will always trump not showing up.

9. **Ask questions** – Are you unsure of what weight to use? Have a nagging "tweak" that is bothering you? Feeling a little run down? That's what your coach is here for! And not only are they open to your questions; they are more than willing to aid you in whatever way possible.

10. **Make friends -** Innovation Fitness is not a come in, put your headphones on, workout, and go home kind of establishment. We are here to create a positive, supportive environment to keep you accountable when you'd rather eat a pint of Ben and Jerry's and watch Netflix than hit the gym. So, say "Hello!" to the newcomers and stick around to stretch and converse for a few minutes after class.

11. **Pay attention to your Coach -** Don't talk while your coach is talking. All the Achievers are trying to receive instructions, please do your best to minimize or put a pause to personal conversations and sidebars during this time. Resume them when all participants have received their instructions.

12. **Be coachable -** Your coach became a coach to help people become better, stronger, faster, and healthier. Listen to them. Even if the skill they are teaching is a strength of yours, listen anyway. You just might learn something new, and the day we stop learning is the day we stop excelling.

13. **Never say, "I can't" -** Learning new skills and getting good at them takes time. Saying, "I can't" isn't going to help you get stronger or improve your execution. Have patience and try not to get frustrated. Know that improvement is a process.

14. **Put form before all else -** Put your time and energy into perfecting your form and your overall potential to increase strength while staying safe will increase. Conversely, if you just go through the motions or lift with your ego instead of your brain, you will increase your risk of injury and end up missing training time. Training is a humbling experience. No matter how strong, fast, tough you are, at the end of the workout everybody looks the

same laying on the floor in a pool of sweat. Don't cover up your vulnerability, own it. This is what makes you human.

15. **Look to improve daily -** Practice equals progress. Pick a skill and make it your prerogative to get good at it. Dedicate a few minutes before and after a session to develop this skill and before you know it, you will own an additional strength.

16. **Be on time -** From time to time, life gets in the way and lateness cannot be avoided. However, consistently arriving 15 minutes prior to the start of the session is a terrific way to mentally prepare to be at your best and physically prepare your body via properly warming up.

17. **Always finish your workout -** The only thing between you and finishing a workout is the little voice in your head telling you, you can't. Your Coach will modify anything that needs to be, to keep you safe and progressing, but copping out and cutting things short only hurts your results.

18. **Cheer for Others -** The positive support and camaraderie between our members is a special bond. Everyone wants to do their best and wants the best for the person working next to them. Give a little cheer now and then. It will make the time spent more positive and boost your performance.

19. **Stay involved -** Do your best to attend our events and get-togethers. Join our Social Media outlets and lend your voice with opinions, suggestions, and advice for others. Be just as open to receiving advice and commentary from others.

20. Have Fun! – You are doing something wonderful for your confidence and long-term health. Be proud of your accomplishments, work hard and have a few laughs.

I take total responsibility for my health and my results (Food, Fitness, and Focus). I understand that everyone has issues, which I will treat as obstacles that might take me on a different fitness path, not barriers that will prevent me from reaching my goals.

I understand true health and wellness is about the continued journey, not about reaching a short-term goal. I understand my current physical condition is my fault and no one else's, and only I have the power to change myself. I acknowledge that with proper coaching and by remaining coachable I will be much more likely to achieve and maintain my ultimate success. I also understand my health, physical condition and wellness is the most valuable thing I own and that I have to invest in myself regularly to live my life at a higher level of well-being. I will commit to do the work necessary to create change and I understand that what I put into this endeavor is what I will get out of it.

1. Is there **ANYTHING** that your Coach needs to know to tailor the session to your needs (fatigue, illness, mindset, previous or existing injury)?
2. Have you **EATEN** a snack or meal 60 – 90 minutes prior to the training session? Are you properly **HYDRATED**? Are you continuing to drink consistently during the workout?
3. Did you arrive 10-15 minutes early or the session to **WARM-UP** by using the cardio equipment and light flexibility exercises?
4. Are you **MENTALLY PREPARED** to work hard and are you in the best mood possible? Are you prepared to leave in an even better mood?
5. Are you monitoring your **WELL BEING** during the session, communicating with the Instructor if you feel faint, overly-fatigued, dizzy and/or nauseous?
6. Are you working to your current **SKILL LEVEL** and physical ability? Be intelligent about your exertion and challenge yourself, but do not put yourself into a position of injury.
7. Do you agree to be **CONSISTENT**? Making your attendance a priority and not making excuses, but instead finding solutions to live a Fitness Lifestyle will bring you closer to your goals.

Fitness Guide

FITNESS DISTINCTIONS

Fat Loss > Weight Loss
Lifestyle > Dieting
Nutrition > Calories
Quality > Quantity
Strength > Cardio

Results are not linear
Food is information
Metabolic Compensation
Shades of Grey
Measure What Matters

Principles and Distinctions

Know your "WHY"

Before deciding on anything else in your new lifestyle, it is imperative to tie your goals to an anchor. My experience with many clients has shown a few things to be crystal clear – one of these is the people that know WHY they are making changes are much more likely to remain consistent and overcome obstacles and setbacks as they arise. These people are tied to something much bigger and more meaningful than "just" losing weight. They have a vision for their life. During times of stress or diversion, they remain keenly aware that setbacks and missteps are part of the change process and that they will recover because they NEED to stay true to their anchor. Your WHY is your driving force. My own experience and my guiding force for my decisions stem from my desire to be the best role model for my two sons that I possibly can be. This position and this REASON are the place that my decisions emanate. Picture your life and your choices tied to a REASON. When I am under duress and potentially unsure of what to do, if I am feeling "lazy" and am actively looking for an excuse to allow myself to skip exercise or make a poor food choice or act in a reactive way that may be harmful to myself or a relationship, that guiding anchor drives my decisions and allows me to make a better choice. I am first and foremost a role model to my sons. Picture a scenario where you have a driving force and find it. Make your choices from that place, based upon those reasons

You need to ask yourself...

Why does fat loss matter to me?
Fat loss isn't the goal. The goal is how you'll feel once you've lost fat.

The takeaway? Fat loss is not the goal. The goal is how you will feel once you have lost fat.

This "why" is what pushes you to persevere through the tough workouts and hunger pangs to stay the course.

Dig deep and find out the "why" behind your motivation. You will not always like what you find, but it is what you need to do to lose fat and keep it off.

Programming Fat Loss

Introduction

Sustained fat loss is challenging to say the least. There are quick fix plans, social media "gurus" and an indoctrinated diet culture to overcome as well as impatience, a lack of scientific competency and peoples' low self-esteem to battle. All is not lost You can change your life for good.

With that, it is primarily lifestyle choices that we can discuss here – mindset, planning, preparation and follow-through is more than enough to help you make the changes they want in their lives.

Here is the list of non-negotiables we need to create to provide a functional and sustainable program.

- Create an 'honesty covenant' so there is accountability and truthful conversations.
- Create an emotional attachment to what they want (Their WHY).
- Properly set goals (outcome and habit goals) (Their WHAT)).
- Together, create a plan that you can perform and repeat. (Their HOW)
- Learn the difference between fat loss and weight loss.
    - All weight loss is not good weight loss. All weight gain is not bad weight gain.
    - Calories have more than one destination.
- Assess your personality type to find which type of programming you will respond best to (Lifestyle vs Short-term Assault).
- Learn to measure what matters. Teach them what to measure for their results, when to measure it and how to measure it.
    - Simply, it is not just about weight loss and how fast you can lose it.
- Learn the scientific laws of weight control repeatedly in different and creative ways.
- Ask yourself challenging questions.
- Learn to strengthen your "patience muscle" daily.
- Ensure that you know that their food choices are OUTCOMES.
    - First, you think and feel things, then you make choices.
- Utilize a complete, WHOLEistic approach to programming that includes calories, stress management, sleep, hydration, training periodization and recovery.

Where do you start?

There is an order to successful fat loss programming.

1. Uncover deep, meaningful goals and reasons for changing (Why)
2. Set outcome and habit goals (What)
3. Decide on the programming style (How)
4. Develop a realistic and sustainable plan of action (How)
5. Educate on and prepare the client for setbacks, plateaus, and achievements. (Coach)

Reverse Engineering – Setting Goals that Work

During an initial meeting, clients tend to give outcome-based goals that lack meaning, direction, or a chance for course correction. "I want to lose X # of pounds" generally covers the extent of goal-setting discussions.

Digging a bit deeper and minimally, setting a timeline to the goal is helpful. "I want to lose X # of pounds in X # of months." Will allow you a glimpse that their perception of themselves, their abilities and how grounded they are.

Deeper still is a layer of goal setting related to not just what they want, but, more so, WHY they want it. When we can have the client illuminate their deep emotional connection to why the above goals are so important to them, this is when we, as Coaches can begin to have our biggest impact.

Reverse engineering – what is it? Basically, it is starting at the goal and working backwards to create the steps it will take to achieve the goal.

Example –

In 2001, while Eldrick "Tiger" Woods was winning just about everything on the PGA Tour, he released a book titled 'How I play Golf'. There were numerous, incredible insights in this book, and it is to this day, a great read, worthy of your time. In it, Tiger describes how he approaches each hole of a golf course. Yes, you guessed it, by reverse engineering the hole.

Most of us, when we play Golf, besides improving our CPM (curses per minute) rate, take out a Driver at the start of each hole, hit it as hard and far as we can (hoping it goes straight(ish) and then dealing with the next shot based on where the first shot came to lie. Tiger, unlike us mortals starts from the green and works back to the tee box.

Where is the flagstick today?

How does the green undulate where the flagstick is?

Where is the best placement for my golf ball on the green based on where the flagstick is?

Which club and type of shot will get me closest to this spot?

Maybe, for Tiger it is a 125-yard wedge into the green, lofted high with moderate backspin. His next question would be – which club do I need to hit off the tee box to put me in that position? If it is a 425-yard Par 4 golf hole, his Driver may go too far with a full swing, hence, throwing his plan off and diminishing his chances of success. So, he may need to hit a 300-yard 3-wood to get him in the correct position.

This is reverse-engineering. Working from the goal backwards to create the plan.

How do we implement (RE) for fat loss programming?

First, we need their WHY. It is what ties this whole program together. Without why, we simply have a bunch of WHAT's… Here is an example from an actual client in her 50's just beginning her journey.

WHY = EMOTIONAL DRIVER Active, BADASS Grandma	
OUTCOME GOALS - WHAT	**OUTCOME GOALS - WHAT**
Lose 20 pounds	Perform 1 Chin-up
Fit in smaller size clothing	Able to get to the floor and back up fluidly.
Happier looking in the mirror	Able to run and play for 20 mins without stopping.
Feel confident in a dress	Confident enough in my body to hike and go skiing
Feeling confident in my sexuality	Laugh more and be less stressed

Some of these goals are subjective, so you will need to organize how you will know when the goal has been attained. Others are objective, making the realization simple. Another observation may be the realization that many of these goals are performance based, not just weight loss based. To me, this is a sign of great coaching – when you realize that you can be more and want more than just a scale #. You may have been convinced that you started this journey so you could lose 20 pounds. The realization that this is part of your goal - a small part of what you want and that it may only be part of what must happen to get to your actual goals is clarifying, inspiring and exciting.

Once you have the WHY and the WHAT's, it is time to discuss the details – the HOW (Plan). I utilize the "Pirate Map" made popular by Dan John. It is a simplified, step by step list of actions. I generally break them up into a daily and a weekly routine.

DAILY MAP	WEEKLY MAP
Drink 16 oz more water per day	Strength train 3 times
Strive to eat vegetables twice+ daily	Go for a walk 3x + if possible
Take my multi-vitamin	Read for 20 mins 3x +
Perform my 5 min stretches twice daily	Gratitude journaling 3x+

What you can take away from this mapping sequence is that the emotional driver uncovers the motivator, which leads you to uncover multiple meaningful goals and helps you create her programming. See how each of the actions lends itself to achieving the goals? The goals and actions need to be discussed and selected by you and the client as a doable, achievable, and sustainable current program. Once these new habits take hold, or goals are achieved, programming must evolve. Obviously, this is not all that needs to be performed to attain all these goals. The next section will clarify why it is written as it was.

Process vs Protocol – The personality test

Selecting the style and pacing for your clients programming.

One of the first questions I use with clients when we discuss their desire to lose weight is – Would you prefer slower but more sustainable fat loss or quicker but not as sustainable? As a surface question, a typical immediate response is quick and sustainable, which was not one of the options stated for a reason…

Following up on this question –

After you discuss the options of quicker results but giving some of those results back (not an option) or taking a slow, habit-focused approach, do your best to describe both to help the client choose for themselves which approach will work best. A habit-based approach is gaining competence in one specific habit at a time, such as eating breakfast daily or drinking more water daily or increasing their Protein or Fiber intake. It is an "ownership and layering" approach. Own the competence of one thing, then layer another habit on top of that while sustaining the first.

A quicker-paced approach has a deadline, say… 6 weeks. It has more of a protocol to it – do this and this and this every day. This approach will see quicker results because more changes are being performed at once. At the end of the established program, you are "released" from the protocol. In the best case, you adopt and maintains some of the habits to minimize any yo-yo effect. Typically, I will discuss the likelihood of a 25-50% rebound dependent on how you follow-up after the protocol.

There are benefits and drawbacks to each of these styles and the goal is to aid you in choosing the best path. A few questions to ask that might help someone decide their success style –

How often do you attempt to lose weight?

How successful have you been?

What have you done that you feel helped you?

How long did you do it for?

What personality do you possess?

Are you more passive or assertive/aggressive?

Are you extremely busy and have no problem filling every minute of their time?

You see, you may be confused about weight loss and everything that is available. The weight loss industry has become one scheme followed by the next and it has helped our population reach higher and higher bodyweights while aiding in declining our health. You have an opportunity to alter your approach, to see that not only can you lose weight, but, with proper coaching you can achieve this with much simpler, less stressful methods and fewer, less critical self-judgements.

Now, back to pros and cons -

The habit-based approach is slow. It requires patience. Lots of it. It may seem at times that results are stagnant, and this may be a deterrent for some. Contrary, if someone is patient, this method is suitable for astounding, sustainable changes. When I discuss this option with clients, I have them look at a 12 -24-month view. By following this process, in 12 months you will look and feel ______ ______ _____.

The quicker, protocol-based choice sets up more dramatic results. It is certainly more restrictive and requires much more immediate planning and execution. I like to say that this style is much more Type A personality style and is much better suited for intense individuals. As with anything, the more weight/fat that is lost and the more restrictive the protocol, the less of the result you get to keep. That is the trade-off. This needs to be crystalized in the clients' mind.

One of the things we as fitness professionals need to do is to minimize weight rebound by setting follow-up protocols. When my clients choose this path, I let them know that we are doing the initial program for 5-6 weeks, then off protocol for 5-6 weeks. Revisit the protocol for 3-4 weeks, then 6-8 weeks off protocol.

This allow them to be fully invested when it is time to be and relaxed when it is time to be. Framing the reasons why their weight loss program needs to be this way is a vital component of compliance.

Bottom line – Will you be more successful with a habit-based lifestyle approach or more protocol, short-term focused?

Protocol "pirate map"–

It is much more focused and directed.

Week 1-3	
Physical Training	**Nutritional Targets**
5-minute morning Flow (stretches)	Journal food intake for first 2 weeks
10,000 steps daily minimum	Protein at every meal
Strength – Mon Workout #1, Wed #2, Fri #3 Sat or Sun #4	Vegetables at every major meal + snack on Sugar Snap Peas and Carrots
1-minute Plank + 1- minute Bridges + 1-minute R/L Pigeon stretch x3 every evening	Nutrition shake for breakfast
10-minute walk and stretches during lunch break.	96 oz – 128 oz of water daily

FITNESS DISTINCTIONS

Fat Loss > Weight Loss

Lifestyle > Dieting

Nutrition > Calories

Quality > Quantity

Strength > Cardio

Results are not linear

Food is information

Metabolic Compensation

Shades of Grey

Measure What Matters

The order of things –

For a protocol focused individual, teach about calories, then mindful/intuitive eating.

For a process focused client, calories are much less a priority as a lesson. Instead focus on journaling.

DISTINCTION #1

Fat Loss is more important than weight loss

Weight loss stated as a goal is vague and incomplete. Do not get me wrong, people probably do need to lose weight. However, focusing solely on how much total weight is lost is a one-way road to not achieving the type of physical and mental transformation people are truly looking to achieve. Instead, we need to focus on the type of weight being lost (or gained).
All weight loss is NOT good weight loss. All weight gain is not bad weight gain.

FAT LOSS	WEIGHT LOSS
• MINDFULNESS	• MINDLESS
• v CALORIES	• v CALORIES
• ^ NUTRITION	• NO EXERCISE OR CARDIO
• ^ PROTEIN	
• ^ FIBER	
• ^ WATER	
• ^ HIGH VOLUME FOODS	
• = BALANCED HORMONES	
• ^ STRENGTH TRAINING	

Weighing in on weighing in –

Weight Range

Many people are guilty of weighing themselves every day, or even multiple times a day while following a diet and exercise regimen because they want to experience immediate results. However, the effects of changing your eating habits and being more active are not instantaneous. It usually takes a couple of days or weeks before you can see a significant drop in your weight if you follow a healthy diet plan. If you weigh in everyday, there is a big chance that you will be disheartened because of the slow progress when it comes to shedding 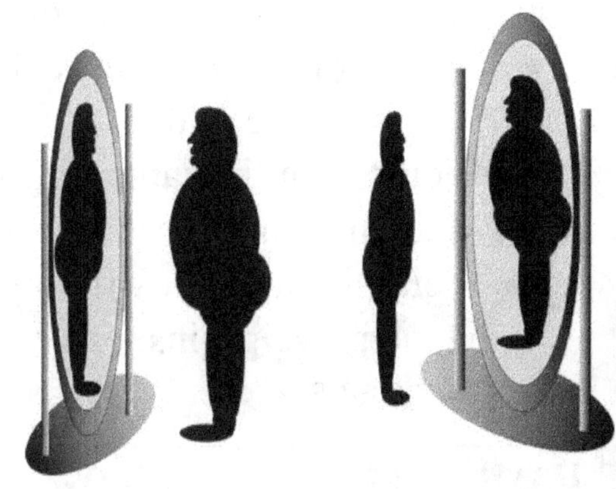 pounds. Additionally, most people do not have a steady bodyweight but, rather, a body weight range. It is normal to fluctuate +/- 2-5 lbs. every few days. This is essential information for a dieter to understand as you are in control of some of the factors that cause the fluctuation and not in control of many others.

Keep in mind that there are 3500 calories in 1- pound of body fat. So, if you gained or lost 2 pounds from day to day it is HIGHLY unlikely that you created a 7000-calorie surplus or deficit to achieve the weight fluctuation.

Scale usage should be utilized for watching your weight trend. The best method is to begin by finding your body weight range. To do this - weigh daily for 5 days and mark the lowest and highest weights. This is your natural body weight range.

As an example, if Monday you weigh 167 lbs., Tuesday 164 lbs., Wednesday 166 lbs., Thursday 167 lbs. and Friday 165 Lbs. Your body weight Range is 164 - 167 lbs. Every time you step on the scale you should expect to see a number in that range.
While creating better food and fitness habits you will lose weight slowly. If you were losing 1-lb. of fat per week your body weight range would shift at the end of 1 month. That means it would go from 164 - 167 lbs. down to 162 - 165 lbs. At least half of the days would be within the lower end of your original BW range.

If scale watching has you in a good mood because the scale moved down or worse... a bad mood because it rose, you need to recheck how you are defining success. The scale will move regardless of how well you are eating or working out. Put the #'s in perspective by understanding the components of body weight (BW). Be aware of your weight range and watch your BW trend for true long-term results. Measure your progress off the range, not the static scale number. *It will not be the same from day to day.*

Tips for Weighing In

After you have found your starting BW range be sure to weigh yourself at least once a week once you get started. To minimize fluctuations, follow these tips for weighing in:

- Wear similar clothing each time
- Use the same scale
- Weigh in at the same time of day
- Maintain similar eating and drinking patterns prior to weighing in
- Weigh in mid-week if you only check your weight weekly
- Monday weigh-ins tend to be inaccurate because of food choices and eating habits on weekends

Day 1	Day2	Day 3	Day 4

Bodyweight Range =

Other Ways to Measure Progress

If you are making progress in at least two of the following areas, you are on the right track:

- Inches lost, Body fat percentage, Clothing size or fit, Energy levels, Positive Mental Attitude, Improved activities of daily living.

Starting Measurement	1st	2nd	Change
Body Weight			
Body Fat %			
Fat Mass			
Lean Body Mass			
Muscle Mass			
Hydration Level %			
Bone Weight			
Waist Size			

DISTINCTION #2

Lifestyle changes will prove better than dieting   ***Personality driven

As previously discussed, most people fail at dieting (95% gain weight post-diet and end up heavier than when they began). The statistics show that people typically start a diet every 3-4 months. That is a large accumulation of failures over the course of a decade or two. No wonder that many are just skeptical and have lost hope. Part of the reason for this is that people just do not know what else to do AND the diet industry makes its money from people remaining ignorant and uninformed.

In the chart here – you can see different types of diets and how they create their energy deficit. There are layers of slick, marketing hype added to each of these, but, fundamentally, diets all have 2 things in common –

1) They create a calorie deficit.
2) They have great marketing campaigns and get you to believe this method is the best solution.

ALL Diets have 2 things in common
1 - Calorie deficit
2 - Marketing gimmick

There are only 3 ways to restrict calories -
1 - TIME (IF, Don't eat past 8 o'clock)
2 - AMOUNT (IIFYM, Calorie Counting)
3 - TYPE (Good vs. Bad, Fattening vs. Fat Burning)

TRUTH - QUANTITY and QUALITY count. ALL foods are fattening and fat burning. Some are healthy, many are not.

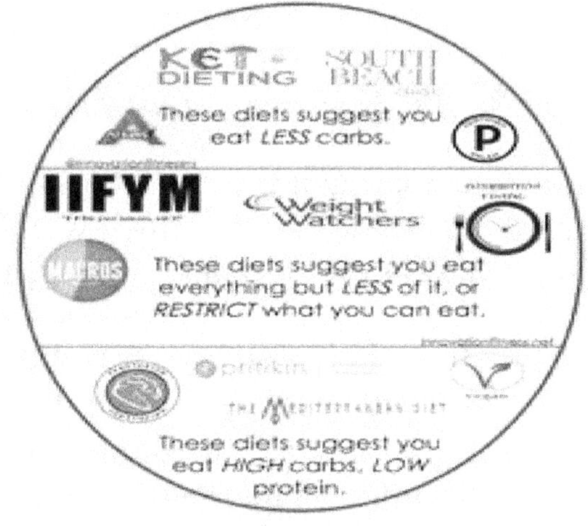

Dieting or diets generally leave the dieter unsuccessful, accumulating failures (which is negative feedback to future attempts) and confused as to what to do next. Add an additional layer of distrust and confusion and the result is an individual that wanders, never gaining traction on changing their habits because they have been conditioned to believe hype and marketing. Simply just waiting for their "next perfect plan" to arrive.

<u>Ownership and Layering.</u> As you gain mastery over one habit and it no longer requires practice and focus, add another. Never before that. In practice, it could be learning to consistently drink more water or gain another hour of sleep, add more vegetables to your intake, to keep a journal or practice stress-reducing techniques.

Lifestyle - Which Fat Loss habits are you currently working on?

Here are examples of habits to implement and track for sustainable results.

Weight/Fat loss is the outcome of many habit changes practiced consistently; it is not a goal.

1) Drinking an adequate amount of water every day?

2) Decreasing liquid calories? *** except #4
3) Ensuring proper Protein intake?

4) Daily Protein Supplement or Meal Replacement Formula?
5) Eating more fruits and vegetables?
6) Planning your meals and mealtimes?

7) Strength training 3-4 times per week?
8) Practicing patience and mindfulness (including slowing your speed of eating)?
9) Keeping a food journal (for accountability purposes) for 2 weeks at a time (every 4-6 weeks)?
10) Increasing daily movement by standing instead of sitting or walking instead of standing or planning 10 minute Workouts in addition to your scheduled gym workouts?

EMPOWERMENT & SUSTAINABILITY

To be <u>POWERFUL</u>, you must first be <u>EMPOWERED</u>.

Often, we approach weight/fat loss as a <u>REACTION</u> to something negative happening or having occurred. I.e.: "I gained weight", or "I didn't get the promotion I deserve", "She lost 20 pounds, now I feel insecure, so I will lose weight too!" or anything, really…

The practice of choosing your response in place of reacting will bring you much more clarity, conviction, and sustainability in the weight loss game (in all of life, really). <u>RESPOND</u>, do not react. Responding to a thought and/or feeling is positive and powerful. Reacting, generally leads to trouble. Remember, it is never one choice that stalls progress, it is the next choice and the next and the next… Borrowing a credo from Alcoholics Anonymous – Logic over Emotion. Responding is logical and allows us to remain in control of our choices. Reacting to fleeting emotions or giving into current thoughts and feelings is the single most hurtful action anyone on a weight loss journey can do because there will always be a life challenge to overcome. If you are reacting, you are in a constant state of defense.

Something that I find vital while working with clients is to do my best to understand where they are in their journey, including their mental makeup. During conversations, providing feedback and validating someone's' thoughts and feelings is supportive and lends itself to gaining trust. Minimizing ones' thoughts and feelings to simply provide a list of "to-dos' and NOT to-do's is the opposite. When I am the most successful with clients it is because I am in a headspace that allows me to see them, what their struggles are, what their resources are and what their current abilities are, this enables me to help connect the dots with them. When I struggle, it usually is due to my impatience in trying to get them to their goal by offering the "to do" list.

- Eat this, not that.
- Do these workouts.
- Follow this specific strategy…
  All of these represent a convenient, short-sighted path to nowhere.

MINDSET MATTERS MOST

As we discuss often throughout this book, a strong and resilient mindset will do more for our wellness efforts than any other single aspect of fitness. Often, though, we will suffer from a "victim mentality", meaning, we believe that outside circumstances are to blame for our lack of progress. Having a mindset that claims ownership of choices and accepts accountability for our actions certainly makes fat loss success easier. Honestly, there is not much anyone can do to help a client that refuses to accept responsibility for their lifestyle. Fortunately, we have tools to facilitate the journey to accountability.

While utilizing a perfectionist mindset, we mistakenly believe that we are holding ourselves to an extremely high standard. A perfectionist mindset is a surefire way to balk at the slightest imperfection that leads to a non-stop cycle of starts and stops.

A healthy mindset allows for mistakes, detours, and slip-ups. It allows us to remember that we are not perfect, that we have failed numerous times at numerous things in life but none of that matters if we do a little bit better in the positive direction than our failures pull us in the negative. A healthy mindset looks at progress, not perfection.

When we assume ownership over the following, we own the ability to create a different lifestyle.

Control
- You control your outcome because you control your environment.
- You control the thoughts you think and the actions you take.
- You control what you eat or do not eat and how much you eat or do not eat.
- You control how much you move or do not move.
- You control your excuses or actions.

Past lessons can be useful tools to see where you have gone wrong and to utilize that information to inform you about what does and does not work for your life.

Many popular weight loss programs include substantial information about nutrition, food, exercise, and meal plans, but fail to address aspects of lifestyle. If the miracle diet pill, book, exercise program or video worked so well then why do we gain our weight back so often? My research tells me that it is all these reasons:

1. **You were not ready to commit to a different lifestyle.**
2. **You did not know how to get started and stay on the right track.**
3. **You lacked the proper education necessary to make the change stick.**
4. **You wanted a quick fix.**

<u>Failure leaves clues.</u> The 3 most common things people consistently struggle with their weight (or any area of their life) are these –

1. "All or None" Mindset

Many people in life (not just weight loss endeavors) adopt and hold true to the mindset of PERFECTIONISM or "All or None". This mindset shows itself in numerous ways, but most often, it rears its ugly head during conflict. Many clients I have had are OK if everything is going well. Their choices are sound, their thinking is pure, and their mood is good. However, as soon as one area of life causes stress this creates a spiral of negative thinking and their mindset goes from "I am in control" to "This is not working, I quit!"

The stressor could be a work conflict or poor food choice or a missed exercise session, a bounced check or anything really. This "All or None" mindset makes it increasingly difficult to attain and maintain success because the thought process relies on the foundation of perfection.

A better plan is to understand that negative situations happen to everyone and will happen to you on occasion. Learn to handle stress with proper perspective and gain the ability to understand that every choice counts towards achieving your goal or delaying it.

2. Failing to Plan

A second pitfall I often see is that many people do not plan their meals and workouts. Many people wait for motivation to strike before they act. This is the exact opposite of what needs to be done to gain success.

- You must schedule your workouts as a "**non-negotiable priority**" and attend these important appointments with yourself.
- You must plan and schedule your meals in advance. If you wait until you get hungry to think about what you are going to eat you increase your risk of making poor food choices and eating items that are not in your plan. This may lead to a loss of control (see "All or None").

3. Lacking Consistency

Often, individuals begin a plan when they become distressed about their health, appearance and/or fitness levels. They make multiple drastic changes at once in an all-out effort to achieve as much as possible as quickly as possible. Generally, repeating mistakes from their past. When we attempt to accomplish everything at once in addition to the busy schedule we may already have, we tend to become overwhelmed, ceasing a few of the more important actions of attaining your goal.

Consistency is accomplished by placing priority on the actions that are the most vital for your desired outcome and continuing these actions. You cannot get to your goals with a "tomorrow" attitude.

Knowing the failure of your past methods and agreeing to not repeat them is a vital step in attaining lifelong health. So, included are steps to ensure success and keep failure at bay

What does a healthy weight loss plan look like?

Healthy weight loss is a way to reduce the amount of body fat while preserving your lean tissues. It is a slow and sustained process of altering your way of thinking and your choices to align with your new goals and values of improving and sustaining long-term health.

A healthy weight loss plan provides nutrition for your body and movement to energize you to feel your best. It is an eating style that includes foods, it does not eliminate them from your intake. It is an active lifestyle that gives you fuel and energy to live your best life.

- Healthy weight loss focuses on healthy patterns.
- Healthy weight loss focuses on the long-term outcomes, not instant gratification.
- Healthy weight loss allows for flexibility in your eating, not rigidity and perfectionism.
- Healthy weight loss allows for setbacks and occasional missteps. It does not provide punishment for a poor choice or temporary loss of focus.
- Healthy weight loss is slow and steady, allowing you to feel good about yourself and know that you are making fabulous changes and additions to your life, not sacrifices.
- Healthy weight loss allows you to eat out at restaurants, not sit home alone obsessed with following a "diet".
- Healthy weight loss includes strength training to boost your metabolism, help your posture and allow you to enjoy more food.
- Healthy weight loss is balanced. Healthy weight loss is intelligent and planned, it avoids fads and falling for "miracles".
- Healthy weight loss is a way of life. Your new life.

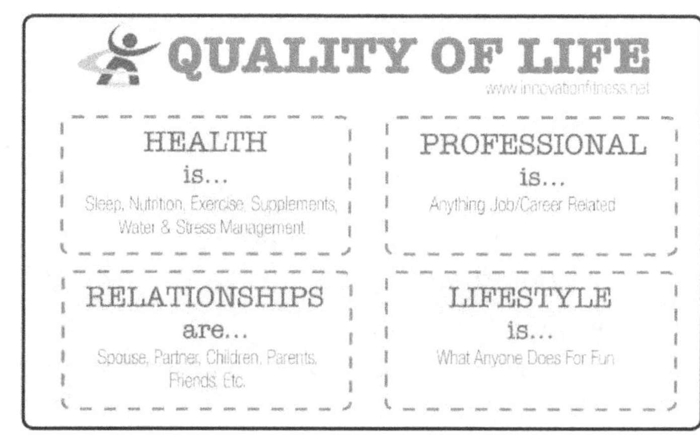

In this new life, you would:
- Know that you have control over many things but do not have control over everything.
- Focus on obtaining fruits, veggies, fiber, and protein from your food choices.

- Focus on moving more simply for the sake of increasing activity.
- Focus on reading and learning to build your "brain muscle".
- Focus on trying new recipes and finding activities to do with your family and friends.
- Focus on your relationship with yourself and with others.

Everything Affects Everything

From the **Mindset Matters Most** section, we are able to see how mood, fatigue, core beliefs and limiting beliefs drive our behaviors. **Everything Affects Everything** allows us to see how weight gain, as unintentional as it may be, is a result of our choices, and how those choices are a direct result of our lifestyle which is a direct result of our priorities, beliefs and actions.

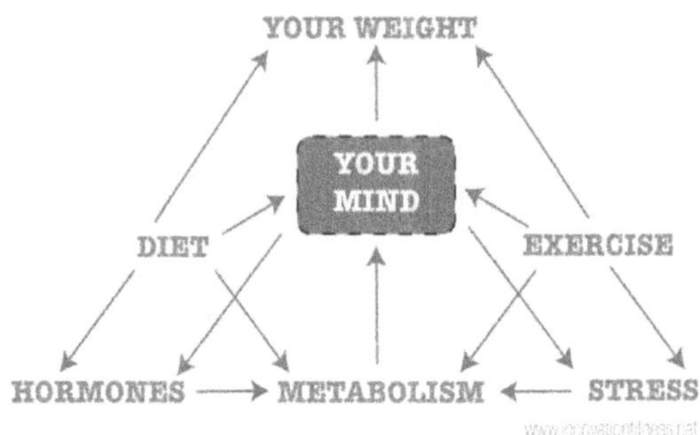

The Calories IN vs Calories OUT **(CICO)** model of weight loss is inarguable, as it is based on the Laws of Thermodynamics, however it is not as simple as "Eat less and Move More", recent studies have uncovered multiple factors that affect metabolism. The diagram above shows that calorie intake can be positively or adversely affected by things like the amount and intensity of stressors, sleep amount and quality, mood, financial stress, what and how much you eat as well as how much and the intensity of movement. Metabolic changes can trick you into eating more even though you may not be hungry. This, in turn, may cause a negative mindset shift and cause greater sabotage to your weight loss efforts.

The mindset side of life has a direct result on our calorie expenditure because when we feel good, we are more likely to move more and more often as well as make food choices aligned with our values that represent the healthy and good in us.

- Many people get stuck either desperately attempting to eat less food/calories for as long as possible or exercising their way thin. Not only is it short-sighted, it is also incomplete.
- Knowing that food choices affect hormones and hormones affect food choices is an important lesson too.
- Knowing that Metabolism is simply the number of calories burned per day and that this is a dynamic figure (not static, as in 2000 calories per day, every day) is also vital to long-term success.
- Knowing that mood, sleep quantity and quality as well as the ability to remain calm all also affect weight gain is an important lesson.
- Knowing that it is not only the quantity of food that causes a scale shift (Up or Down) but, quality also plays a role is vital.
- Knowing that the type, amount, and intensity of exercise impacts the metabolism, affects hunger, and has mood altering abilities is a worthy lesson too.

Even when we clearly understand the physical aspects of transforming our bodies, it is the mind that allows us to veer off course. Putting the following steps into practice, then, becomes a crucial step in creating a powerful and empowering mindset.

1) The ability to delay **INSTANT GRATIFICATION**
    a. The ability to respond instead of reacting to thoughts/feelings/emotions.
    b. A long-term view of health and wellness.
    c. Minimizing the critical nature of diets.
    d. Allowing for "mistakes", missteps, and imperfections.

2) A **POSITIVE SUPPORT SYSTEM**
    a. Individuals besides themselves that lend support in ways that the client responds to and that genuinely have their best interest at heart.

3) **SPECIFIC ACTIONS.**
    a. Not all paths lead to the same place
    b. Weight Gain is typically accidental.
    c. Weight/Fat Loss is intentional.

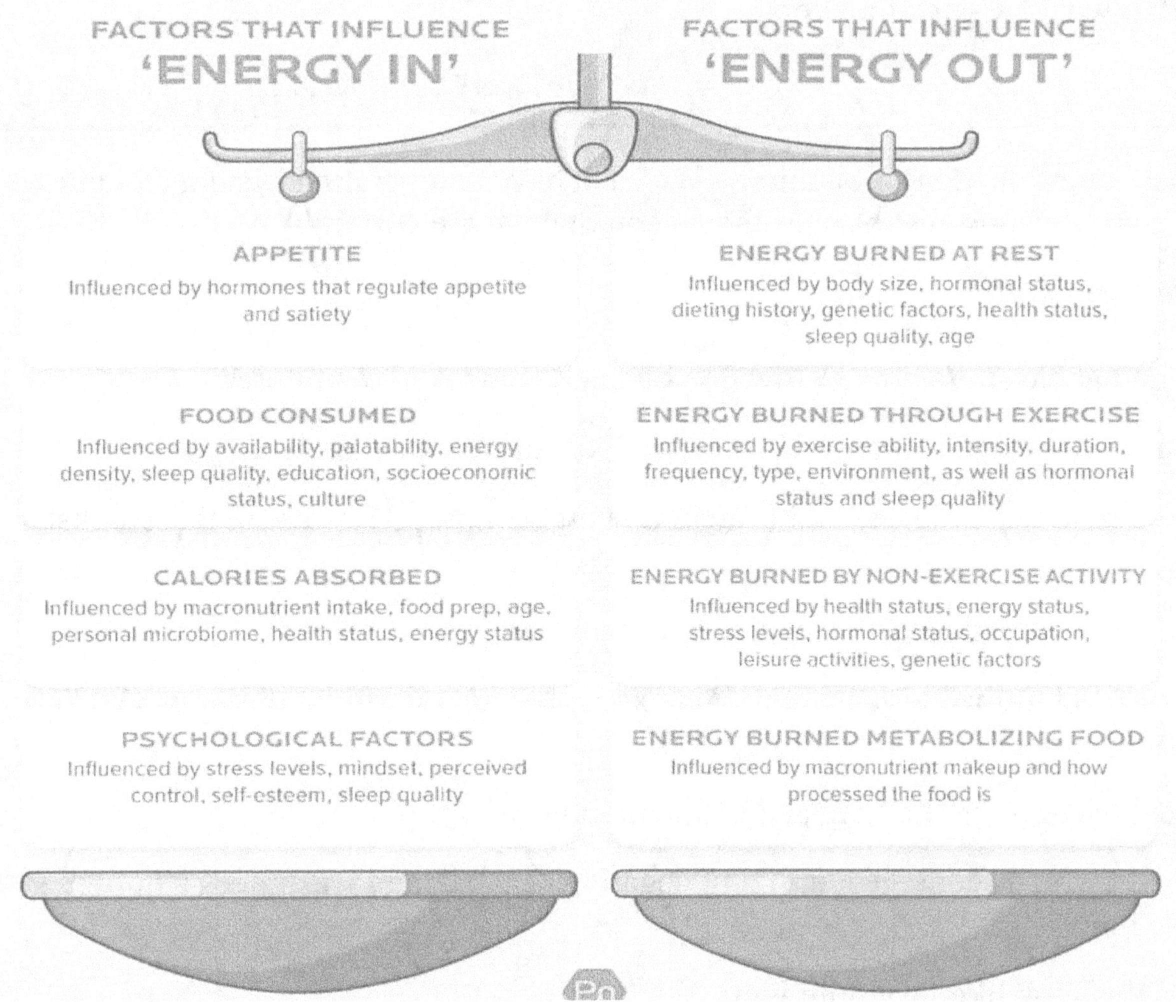

Shades of Grey (Context matters)

Compared to what?

I utilize this question more often than just about any other in my arsenal. Often, we will get frustrated with the pace of progress or fall back into older habits and mindsets that leave us confused and potentially sabotaging our efforts. **Compared to what?** is a simple, direct question that just about immediately (if not sooner) takes us from our "black or white", "all or none", "good or bad" mindset back to patience and focus on progress.

Compared to what? allows for shades of grey. When understood and utilized, it is a relief to not have to constantly fixate on being perfect for fear of any misstep spelling certain disaster, this question creates the possibility of a range of options and outcomes.

Ex: Eating 2 cookies and deciding that you are done may be much better than many previous cookie binges. Many people would get disheartened because they had a cookie or two, forget that they are in process and that they have actual proof of progress by eating less cookies. Perfectionism is the enemy of progress. Most of us have a perfectionist mindset so engrained that any mistake or misstep will damn near guarantee a failure to succeed.

Compared to what? Context matters.

Who do I need to become in order to get what I want?

The ultimate question, don't you think? We each have an operating system that allows us, enables us, and demands us to act as the person that we are currently.

Change talk questions -

How do you handle stress now? How do you handle stress in the future?

How often do you exercise now? How often does future you exercise?

How many servings of veggies and Protein do you eat now? How about that Rockstar – Future you?

How strong is your patience muscle now? Future you?

How often do you utilize justifications and excuses to get out of doing things you know you need to do? Future?

Do you apply rigidity in thinking and application now? Future?

How often are you discouraged, utilizing negative self-talk and frustrated with life? How do you handle it now?

What does this look like for future you?

Results are NOT linear

An ideal scenario sees us make a singular decision and magically maintain the power and ability to repeat it. Reality, however, works differently. Weight loss is not one, single decision, it is a culmination of hundreds of decisions made daily and repeated for infinity.

Most diets are sold on the belief that a protocol, once followed, delivers results that are forever… duh… The issue is that most of us buy into diets at a time of emotional weakness, falsely believing that the result we achieve is the result that will stay.

We know that the body is an adaptive machine (which is illustrated below in 'Metabolic Compensation', so our job needs to be figuring to stay on course when we are fatigued or impatient.

Weekly weight loss goal	Daily calories to reduce or burn through activity
½ lb	250
1 lb	500
1.5	750
2	1000

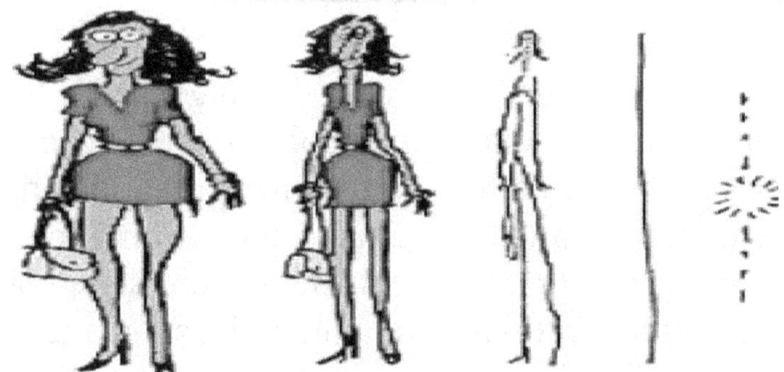

Based on the "classic" calorie deficit model, if you create a calorie deficit and multiply it by time, you will reach your weight loss goal, so long as the deficit is maintained, by this measure, if you kept dieting, you would eventually disappear. There is more than enough evidence to show that chronic, repeated dieting results in long-term weight gain, not loss, which leaves me to believe that there is more to it than a simple calculation. <u>If just eating less and/or exercising more did work, there would never be a need for another diet protocol.</u>

Further, all systems in this Universe work the same way. When we understand in our heart, not just logically, that there will be ups and downs, twists, and turns and that the scale will move up and down frequently, pressure for perfection gets relieved. This may result in us not self-sabotaging nearly as frequently. Delaying the frequency and intensity of setbacks, not eliminating them will bring our ultimate success.

In the 'Measure What Matters' section, there is a list of Physical measurements that I think create a more complete picture of success. There is also a list of mental/emotional measurements that will tell you the real story of how the client is handling life at the present time.

One thing is certain – results vary in all life phases all the time.

Scale weight fluctuates 2-5 lbs. daily, stressors are higher at times, hormonal changes, sleep pattern disruptions, energy spikes and dips, food quality and changes in amount, bowel movement pattern changes all lead to normal and expected fluctuations.

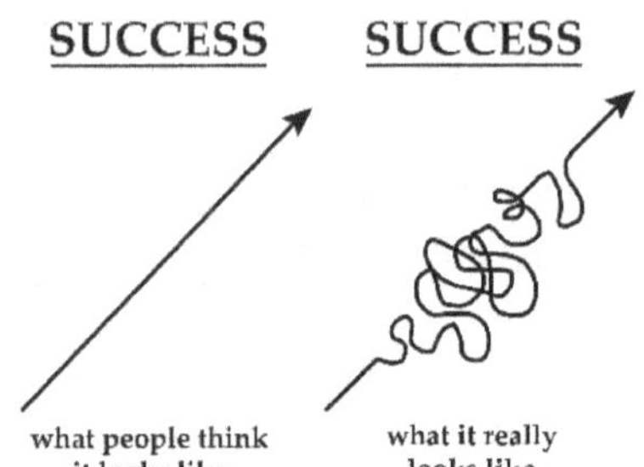

Metabolic Compensation

The body has one single job – survival.
This is seen in the adaptive and reactive nature of metabolism. The metabolism seeks balance or homeostasis. As a result, when you push on the metabolism in any direction, it will push back against you. So, how do you learn to work with the body instead of against it?
You can do this with your metabolism by learning a different strategy than "eat less, exercise more."

- What happens when you eat less? You get hungry, your energy crashes, and cravings ensue.
- What happens when you exercise more (longer, harder, or more frequently)? You get hungry, your energy crashes and cravings ensue.

Not only will it compensate with changes in hunger, cravings, and other sensations, but it will also slow the metabolic rate. This decelerated metabolic output aspect of compensation is known as "adaptive thermogenesis." In other words, through various mechanisms, the metabolism will reduce its rate of caloric burn significantly. Some research suggests up to a 25% decline in daily energy expenditure. These changes seem to be coming from a combination of muscle mass loss, changes in leptin/thyroid output, and a spontaneous decrease in non-exercise associated movement (NEAT).

To beat the metabolism at this game requires you to be diligent with your approach. Not going to extremes with diet and exercise, cycling the approach with periods of less food and exercise for periods of more food and exercise, and learning to read the body's metabolic signals are important strategic maneuvers for metabolic success.

How can you reconcile when to eat less and when to eat more?
First, acknowledge you cannot diet forever. There will always be some metabolic adaption when trying to lose fat. But when fat loss comes to a screeching halt you have two options:
Second, incorporate refeed meals. By increasing the amount of food you are eating you'll increase leptin levels to boost your metabolism and give yourself a mental break from dieting.

Third, reverse diet back to maintenance calories. Reverse dieting is the process of increasing your calories over time to minimize fat gain and repair your metabolism following a diet. If you are coming out of a long-term diet and looking to maintain weight loss, reverse dieting is likely your best option.

Here is a sample:

Maintenance Calories: 2550
Fat Loss Diet Calories: 1650

Reverse Diet Week One:1800 Calories
Week Two: 1950 calories
Week three: 2100 calories
Week Four: 2250 Calories
Week Five: 2400 calories
Week Six: 2550 Calories

The research:
A study published in the *Journal of the American College of Nutrition* in April 1999 showed just how damaging the weight loss model can be on metabolic efficiency. This study looked at a group of obese individuals who were put on a very low-calorie diet and assigned to one of two exercise regimes. One group did aerobic exercise (walking, biking, or jogging four times per week) while the second group did resistance training three times per week and no aerobic exercise.

At the end of the twelve-week study, ***both groups lost weight*** but the difference in muscle vs. fat loss was striking. The aerobic group lost 37 pounds over the course of the study. The resistance-training group lost 32 pounds. A focus on weight loss would lead us to the conclusion that aerobic exercise is best. However, when looking at the type of weight lost it was shown that the aerobic group lost almost 10 pounds of muscle on average while the resistance training group lost fat exclusively and maintained their muscle mass. Most important, when the resting metabolic rate of the participants was calculated, the aerobic group was shown to be burning 210 fewer calories at rest per day!! In contrast, the resistance-training group increased their metabolism by 63 calories per day.

Takeaways? The body strives for efficiency and we must provide a constant state of inefficiency. Higher metabolic rates are inefficient and are accomplished by strength training. Strength Training is the key to altering our clients' appearance and increasing their daily expenditure (resting and exercise-induced).

The avoidance of plateaus is accomplished through progressive overload in strength training, consistently improving food quality while controlling excess energy intake and ensuring that the body has everything it needs to strive except for calories (nutrients/supplements, water, rest, positive stress).

Metabolic Compensation is real and is easy for most of our clients to experience. For the most part, through chronic dieting, they are now able to gain weight eating low-calorie, low nutritional intake while performing cardio exercise. Truly, a recipe for poor health, low performance, and weight creeping.

Weight gain is accidental. Weight loss is intentional. Continual assessments and modifications will be necessary to maintain progress.

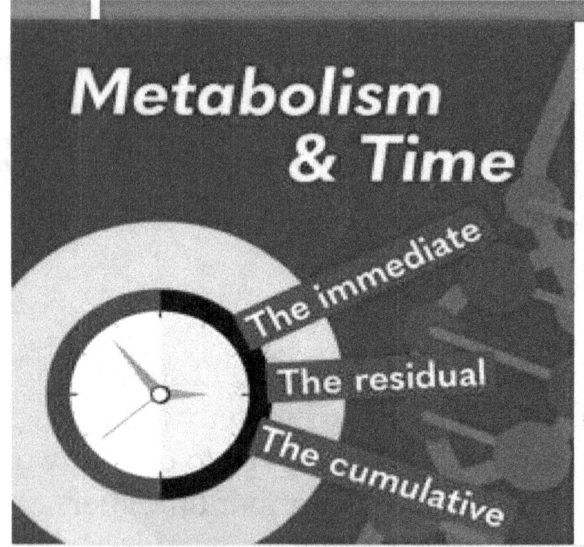

Nutrition > Calories

Nutritional targets are much simpler and more effective than calorie counting

Rather than giving our clients full menu plans, or <<GASP>> having them do the calorie counting thing… we focus our effort towards 3 simple nutritional targets – Protein intake, Fiber intake and Water intake. These 3 things seem to check a lot of boxes and consistent execution seems to accelerate fat loss for most people.

	Minimum	Ideal	Optimal
PROTEIN	.5 oz. / lb BW	.75 gr / lb BW	1.00 gr / lb BW
FIBER	25 grams / day	30 grams / day	35+ grams/ day
WATER	.5 oz. / lb BW	.75 oz. / lb BW	1.00 oz. / lb BW

Reconciling this approach with the calorie model (as suggested above)

In the Metabolic Compensation section, I suggest reverse dieting as a useful strategy, complete with caloric intake suggestions. Caloric intake is the **WHAT**, Nutritional Targeting is the

HOW. Just adding more food will not suffice. The type of food (quality and macronutrient) is vital to successful transformation.

Food is information: Some foods and food combinations make us feel energetic, light, and help to control our energy, hunger, and cravings. Others make us feel awful. Whether it be an insensitivity or an allergy. Learning to utilize more of the foods that fill us, satisfy us and help us minimize uncontrolled eating will help us to reach and maintain our goals.

If we were to poll our clients with a question – **What is Food?** Most would probably immediately answer along the lines of food is calories or food is energy. When taken to another level, food is information to the body and your mind. Food can create powerful memories of the past (good or bad) provide comfort or be a source of stress and fear. Food can be a source of joy (social, celebratory) or it can be a source of feelings of failure (not following protocol, breaking a diet).

To say that food is nothing more than calories, or, just as popular and just as incomplete – food is fuel is a disservice to the power that food plays in each of our clients' lives. Part of our job as Coaches needs to center on helping the client to understand their relationship with food. The information is present, we simply need to help them uncover the patterns and feeling they associate with eating.

Quantity is important, BUT quality is <u>important-*ER*</u>

Weight Gain and loss is controlled by your quantity of food calories over a long period. Your health, leanness and tissue quality are controlled by food quality over a long time period. Your workout performance is guided by meal frequency, meal content and macronutrient breakdown which can be felt daily.

For our clients, improving their food quality can be one of the most important and practical practices to work on. It is a fantastic way to increase meal satiety and volume, increase thermic effect of food and improve the state of their health.

Strength training takes priority over adding MORE cardio

Many clients mistakenly believe that metabolism is a static measurement (My metabolism is 2000 calories). We know that sleep quantity and quality affect metabolism, cravings and hunger, we know that mindset directly affects mood which has an impact on food intake and energy expenditure, and we know that movement increases daily metabolism. Strength trainings role in fat loss programming cannot be <u>underscored</u> enough. Training boosts short-term and long-term metabolic rate and it is the stimulus to transform our clients' appearance. Programming wise, Cardio has many more limiting factors than a progressive strength program.

Measure What Matters

"If you can't measure it, you can't improve it." – Peter Drucker

Through the years, I have collected and created numerous methods (Standards, if you will) for measuring meaningful progress. Presented here are charts for Daily, Weekly, Monthly and Semi-annual measurements.

The *daily measurements* can give near real time data in a combination of objective and subjective styles. Stress levels should be at 6 or lower. Sleep hours are to be at 6+ while Hunger levels should be at 6 and below. Energy, we strive for 6+ and Cravings should be at 6 or lower.

These figures represent the minimal necessary environment for change to occur and to maintain as much control as possible. These figures also give you the reasoning as to why you are succeeding or struggling and how to solve for the challenges.

Weekly measurements are designed to prevent weight creeping, build rational thinking regarding scale weight, and provide a non-scale focus to maintain positivity and momentum.

Monthly Measurements are present to show trend lines and actual progress. They serve to give the data needed for program modifications for weight loss, also to celebrate many other goals for improved fitness and health.

Semi-annual measurements are intended to show health improvements and mindset changes.

Daily Measurements

	Stress Level	Sleep (Hours)	Hunger	Energy	Cravings
Mon					
Tue					
Wed					
Thu					
Fri					
Sat					
Sun					

*Adopted and adapted from Dr. Jade Teta

Weekly Measurement

Date	Weight Range	Change

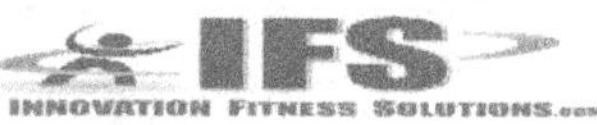

Non-Scale Victories	Gratitude List	Reasons to Smile

Monthly Measurements

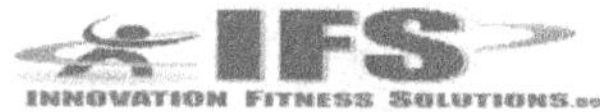

Bodyfat %	Change	Muscle %	Change	Circumference	Change
DATE:				Waist – Other -	
DATE:				Waist – Other -	
DATE:				Waist – Other -	
DATE:				Waist – Other -	
Heart Rate	Change	Heart Rate Recovery	Change	Fitness Test	Change
DATE:				1 Mile Test – BW Strength -	
DATE:				1 Mile Test – BW Strength -	

*** BW Strength Test = 20-minute time limit – Max Reps – Chin-up variation, Pushup Variation, Squat Variation

Blood Pressure	Lipid Profile	Hormonal Changes	Medications
Date			
Date			

Goals Achieved	Goals Altered	New Goals

Putting ALL of this into practice

Autonomy is the result of learning and applying these lessons. Ultimately, our clients learn the ability to choose their negotiable methods and strategies to accomplish the non-negotiable needs for change. Your Coaching is what will uncover their functional strategies.

Where do we go wrong most of the time?
1) Remaining one-dimensional.
Stubbornly measuring weight loss only, instead of muscle gain and fat losses or strength gains. Weight loss is an outcome of better habits, it does not make for an inspiring goal. Besides, when is the last time your client has not been actively trying to lose weight or thinking about starting to try to lose weight?

Change = Change.

TRANSFORM

NON- Negotiable	Negotiable
Disrupting your comfort zone	HOW you disrupt your comfort zone
Intentional Movement	Your form of exercise
Eating in a caloric deficit	The method/diet you use to achieve deficit
Eating Vegetables	The kind of vegetables you eat
Drinking Water	Other non-caloric fluids
Strength Training	Reps/sets/program
Awareness of intake	Type of Journaling
Self-forgiveness & Compassion	Your own style of constructive reflection
Restraint in indulging	The type of indulgences you choose
Accept responsibility for actions/ behaviors	How you stay accountable
Stress Reduction	Techniques – (more sleep, meditation…)

2) Relying on willpower. Setting strict parameters that require perfection and then giving up due to any imperfection. People tend to toggle between under feeling and undereating followed by overeating and over feeling.

3) **Impatience.** Unraveling your current habits takes time. Creating new ones takes even longer.

4) **Confusion leads to repetition.** Because our clients are so confused by media and input from friends and other peoples' "results" they repeat the same patterns from a position of fear.

Solving for these challenges–

- Create an 'honesty covenant' so there is accountability and truthful conversations.
- Create an emotional attachment to what you want (WHY).
- Properly set goals complete and meaningful goals (outcome and habit goals) (WHAT)).
- Create a plan that you can perform and repeat. (HOW)
- Learn the difference between fat loss and weight loss.
    o All weight loss is not good weight loss. All weight gain is not bad weight gain.
    o Calories have more than one destination.
- Be prepared to work on your "patience muscle" daily.
- Own that your food choices are OUTCOMES.
        o First, you think and feel things, then you make choices.
- Utilize a complete, WHOLEistic approach to programming that includes calories, stress management, sleep, hydration, training periodization and recovery.

How can you begin to do this? Self-Belief and Commitment

Make realistic commitments
Fitness will require realistic investments of your time, energy, and will power. Do not make promises you will not keep.

Visualize your success
See yourself as you want to be. Mental imagery can provide numerous benefits, such as enhancing your belief in your abilities to achieve your goals.

Define fitness for yourself
Discover what it means to you to be fit, then create intelligent goals. Define how your life operates and realize the aspects of fitness and living a fit lifestyle that are enjoyable and offer you lifelong rewards. Keep in mind that your definition will differ from others. Find a fitness goal best suitable to *you*.

3 important change questions:

1. A year from now I'm different. What about my life has changed?

2. I really need to change because?

3. But I can't change right now because?

Commit to get and stay fit
When you make a promise, especially to yourself, it is important to keep it. Dedication is important when you want to achieve a goal. Without commitment, fitness will always be something you want, not something you have. Motivation has its place. It can act as a facilitator to change. However, if motivation is what you become reliant on, you create a habit of doing things only when they are convenient, or, when you feel like doing it. Commitment is a different value altogether. Commitment means that you have come to the realization that taking consistent action is imperative to attain your results. Commitment means that you must act even when you do not feel like it. Motivation acts to stimulate in the short-term. Commitment is

what fuels long-term change. Your thoughts lead your actions; therefore, your mindset must be altered consistently to create empowered belief in self and your actions.

Belief is the basis in all action
- Transform your beliefs and you can change your behaviors.
- If you change your behaviors, you can attain the results you are after.
- Attain your results and you transform your life.
- How you think, affects how you feel, and in turn the actions you take.
- Believe in yourself every day.
- Focus on what you want, being fitter, and healthier, rather than how unfit you are.
- Setting realistic goals and having positive expectations will make all the difference.
- Be Solution Based, not Problem Based.
- It is easy to give up. It takes strength, commitment, and dedication to persevere.
- Begin to think about your possibilities – not your limitations.

Believe that YOU must change it
You cannot pass the buck of responsibility and expect to improve. The responsibility of choice belongs to you. Other people will prove to be great assets in your journey, but in the end, you are the one who is going to make it happen. You must want to improve enough to make it your personal mission. You cannot be inconsistent with changes and expect to achieve anything worth having. You cannot be considering it. You cannot even be fairly sure about it. You must be rock solid and committed to the process of change.

Believe you CAN change it
You may have failed in the past, but that does not matter. When you put your mind to it, you can do amazing things. Do you believe that you can lose weight? Once you own the belief that you can, and you will be unstoppable.

Your results are a consequence of your thoughts, feelings, and actions.
Your thoughts are a product of your values, beliefs, and habits.

The R.P.M. Principles

Realistic:

The R simply means that the change must fit your current and NEXT lifestyle. If it does not, you will not keep doing it and will return to your previous habits (see Stages of Transformation pg 41). Choose foods that you enjoy eating and will continue to eat. Choose methods and strategies that allow you to control your calorie intake. Choose a fitness plan that you can and will stick with. The "Perfect Plan" is not particularly good if you will not do it. You are a work in progress. Learning and implementing new skills and tools takes time and patience. Where you are now and what you are capable of will change with time and execution.

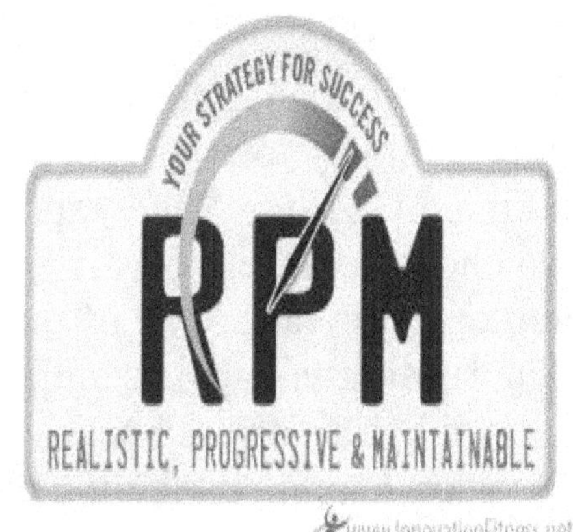

Progressive:

Choose the habits to change that you know you can change. When you "own" those habits, then you can add/layer more. There is no need to tackle everything at once. Do what you can do, not what you can't. A → B then B → C. This method will serve you much better than adopting a "Willpower will win" mentality.

Maintainable:

Success comes from the continuation of habits. Choose against short -term methods for long-term goals. Strategies that you can use daily and repeatedly will always win out over "quick fixes." If you cannot envision yourself doing something consistently, then you are setting up eventual failure. Focus your efforts and reset your thought process. *A → B then C and so on…* You can do something at once, not everything.

Control

- You control your outcome because you control your environment.
- You control the thoughts you think and the actions you take.
- You control what you eat or do not eat and how much you eat or do not eat.
- You control how much you move or do not move.
- You control your excuses or actions.

Consistency

Your results are a product of your habits over time. If you consistently have more good habits than bad ones, then your outcome will be a good one. Consistently strive to do better.

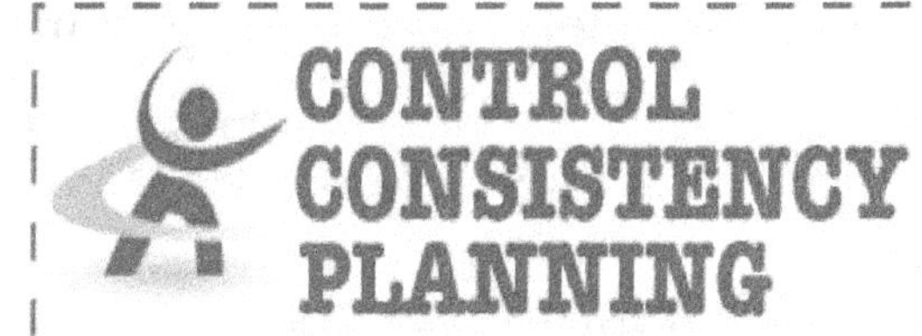

Plan

Planning produces positive performance. If you leave your goals to spontaneity and guesswork, then that will be your result. If you utilize Proper Planning, you will ensure your Positive Performance.

Goals Setting and Expectations

Effectively managing your expectations with realistic short and long-term goal setting is an important key to your success. Many times, we set goals for ourselves that are too aggressive taking an *"All or None"* approach. Although we are overly aggressive from the start, the road we choose is often too difficult to maintain, leading to a viscous cycle of start and stops dieting and exercise fads. One of the most important things that we will accomplish together is determining your goals and creating a clear path for success. Setting short term goals is especially important because long terms goals do not allow us to celebrate achievement along the way, leaving us feeling discouraged.

Expectations

Many times, we set goals for ourselves that are too aggressive. Although we are convinced that this effort will be different, the road we choose is usually too difficult to maintain. This generally leads to the viscous cycle of start and stops dieting and exercise fads. Setting short-term goals is especially important because long-term goals do not allow us to celebrate achievement along the way, thus leaving us feeling discouraged. This book is based on the long-term principle "because you can do it and keep doing it,

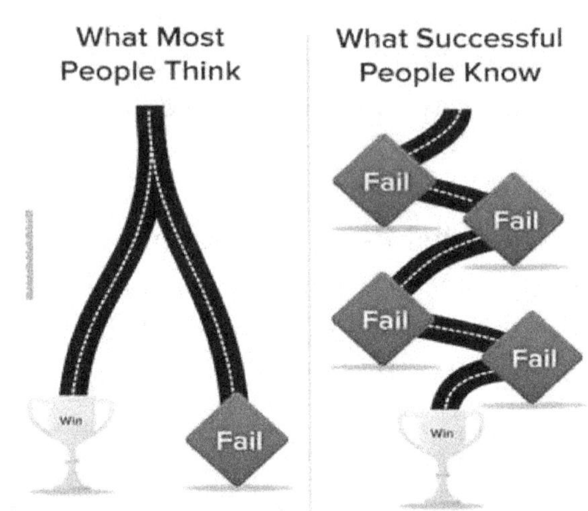

makes it the right plan for you."   You will come to realize that getting to your goals is not as difficult (or as easy) as popular marketing tells you. There is no magic, but it does take planning and consistency. It is not necessary to be so restrictive and hard on you both physically and mentally, but it is necessary to have to expect more from yourself.

Fat Loss vs. Weight Loss

Weight loss does NOT equal fat loss. You may be burning calories or losing weight, but that weight and those calories may or may not be coming from fat. If you follow the standard low-calorie-aerobic-exercise-model, you are likely burning muscle not fat. And a loss of muscle means a less effective metabolism. When individuals focus on weight loss, they are doing a grave disservice to themselves.

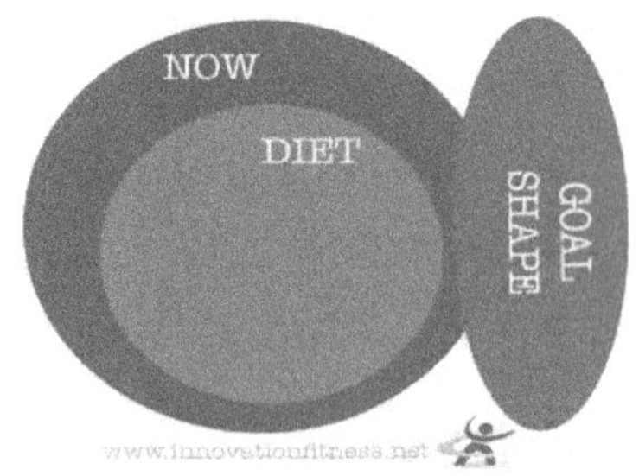

Know the difference between water loss and fat loss.
You will have fluctuations in your weight from day to day. It is important to not get "so happy or excited" when the scale reads a few pounds down and not get "too upset" when the scale is on the high side. Add a bit of logic to this emotional roller coaster. There are 3500 calories in each pound of fat. If you lost 3 lbs. yesterday, did you figure out how to burn 10,500 extra calories? The same

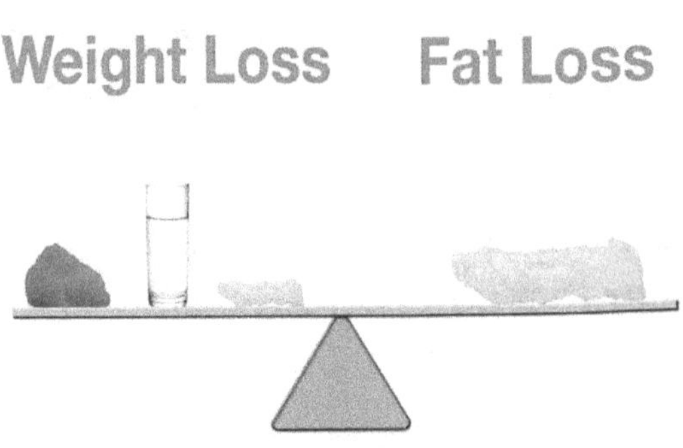

concept applies in the opposite direction. Did you eat 10,500 EXTRA calories yesterday? This fluctuation is normal. Treat it that way.

The calculator vs the thermostat

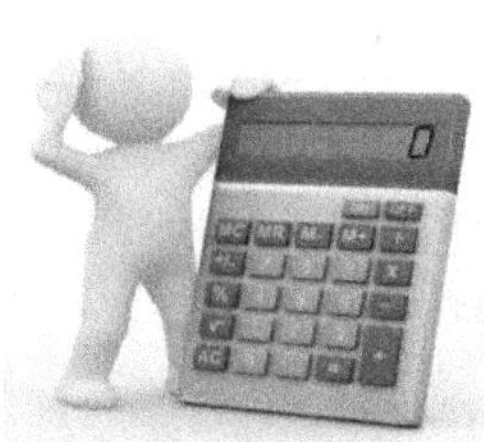

Your metabolism is not like a calculator that responds to a simple formula of addition and subtraction. It's also not like a chemistry lab where you can mix up some defined recipe and get a predictable and repeatable reaction. Your metabolism is more like a thermostat or boomerang. It is an adaptive, reactive system that responds and reacts to everything you do. The job of

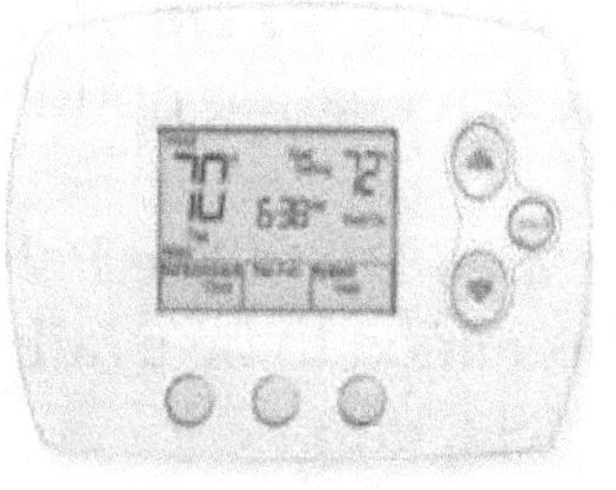

your body is to maintain as much body fat as possible and to make your metabolism efficient.

Quantity and Quality

Consider this - Weight Gain and weight loss is controlled by the quantity of your food calories (How Much) and your health and tissue (muscle or fat) quality is controlled by your Quality (How Healthy). There are plenty of individuals that "Eat Healthy" but cannot budge their weight. This is due to an imbalance of quantity and quality.

If your primary goal is Weight Loss, I suggest controlling your calorie intake and expenditure while eating as many healthy foods as you can stand. Consistently perform strength training to boost metabolic output and change the appearance of your body, not just create a smaller version of yourself. Over time, you will lose weight, have success, and begin to gravitate toward making healthier food choices and creating new exercise habits. Focus on your goal. Perform what you can do and keep doing, not what you feel like you should, but cannot (yet).

The Law of Caloric Restriction

You must restrict calories to trigger fat loss. The most basic rule of fat loss is governed by energy balance. Energy balance is the relationship between energy in, the calories consumed via cheeseburgers (food) and coffee (drinks) and energy out. Energy out is the calories burned through daily energy requirements and exercise. Basically, if you are burning more calories than you're consuming, you should lose weight. This is an oversimplification because the human body is complex. At their root, all successful fat loss diets focus on caloric restriction to drive fat loss.

Examples:

The Slow Carb Diet: The slow carb diet eliminates most starchy carbs, sugars, and fruits to limit the number calories you take in per day.

The Atkins Diet / South beach Diet: The Atkins diet severely limits carbohydrate intake to restrict eating options and drive caloric intake down.

Paleo Diet: The Paleo Diet reflects that of our ancestors and limits food intake to what was assumed to be available in the Paleolithic era (i.e. low carb, only fruits and vegetables; nuts; meat, etc).

Intermittent Fasting: Intermittent fasting limits the amount of time you can eat in a day, making it near impossible to eat too much. There are many other diets and fat loss methods. At the heart of them all is eating fewer calories than your body burns.

The Law of Satiation

Eating a high protein and high fiber diet is a pillar for successful fat loss as protein boosts muscle retention (so your muscles look defined once you are lean) while both fiber and protein keep you full.

What is the secret that makes protein and fiber so important?

Fiber is difficult for your stomach to digest. It takes up a lot of room in your gut and triggers receptors in your brain to tell you that you are full. Even better, fiber slows the release of insulin in your blood stream. So, fiber is a slam dunk which helps you control blood sugar for faster fat loss and gains in lean muscle. Bonus - fiber also improves cardiovascular health, controls diabetes, controls blood pressure, and of course, cleanses your GI tract and give you high-quality poops. ☺

Consuming more fiber does not have to mean consuming more grains. The best weight loss strategy is to replace grains with fiber-rich greens and fruits. At dinner, think about eating steak and asparagus, not a quadruple bacon burger with fries.

What about protein?

Eating a high protein diet is the most crucial factor in improving your physique. For starters, proteins break down into amino acids. These are the powerhouse molecules that replace dead cells, support growth, and help synthesize other important molecules in your body. Eating a high protein diet can boost glucagon, a hormone released when blood sugar drops to stimulate the breakdown of glycogen (stored carbs) into glucose for your body to help you lose stubborn fat. Compared to lower protein diets, high protein diets help you retain lean muscle mass during a diet while also keeping you full.

To maximize fat loss, aim for protein at each meal and aim for at least 1 gram for every pound of bodyweight. To hit your protein goals, eat lean protein like fish, poultry, lean cuts of beef, and mix in the occasional protein shake. Eating protein and fiber rich foods keeps you full and provides your body with essential macros, vitamins, and minerals with fewer calories than most other foods.

The Law of Sustainability

Crash diets are temporary fixes, not long-term solutions.
Crash diets promise massive fat loss in the shortest time possible.
Look no further than the tabloids you see at finer checkout counters everywhere.

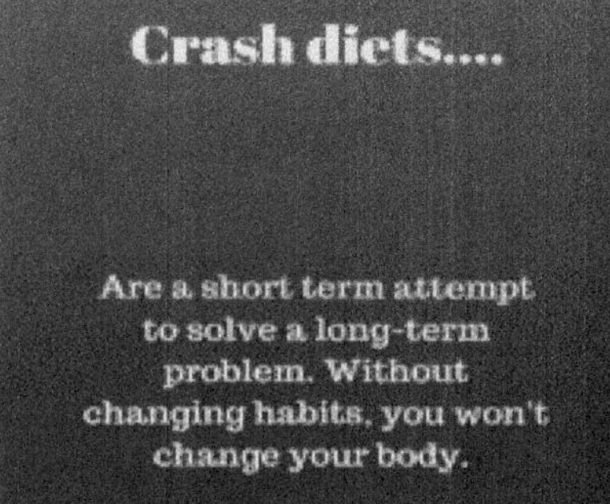

"Lose Ten pounds in Two Weeks!"
"Four Weeks to Fit"

These are catchy headlines, but these are not sustainable methods for lasting fat loss. So, crash diets are useless, right? Not quite. Crash diets work for high-level athletes and physique competitors. It can help them get in tip-top shape. For regular folks, crash diets occasionally work in boosting motivation and building momentum for a diet. But these are the exceptions, not the rule. If you want to lose fat and keep it off, then you need a long-term plan, not a hyped-up band-aid approach. A better approach is recognizing and modifying the behaviors that got you fat in the first place. You cannot crash diet your way into healthy, sustainable habits.

I understand the attraction of following the Grapefruit Diet or whatever shit Gwyneth Paltrow shares on the internet promising 20 pounds off in three weeks. But this is the exact type of yo-yo dieting that leads you to gain and lose the same 20 pounds year after year.

I follow an approach taught by Precision Nutrition, One to One Nutrition and many other professionals, which utilize techniques from Cognitive Behavioral Therapy, Rational Emotive Behavioral Therapy and Neuro-Linguistic Programming to help my clients tweak one small behavior at a time. This builds long-term, sustainable fat loss. Here's a sample six-week approach:

Weeks 1-2: Focus on drinking one glass of water before each meal
- For optimal hydration and to keep you full.

Weeks 3-4: Drink a protein shake after your workout or for Breakfast
- Protein intake is strongly correlated with fat loss and dietary success.

Weeks 5-6: Eat a vegetable with each meal.
- Vegetables are low in calories and high in fiber, vitamins, and minerals to fill you up and give your body the fuel it needs.

Simple? Yes. But simplicity begets consistency, and consistency drives change and fat loss. Ten percent of the time use an aggressive fat loss approach to move the needle and build momentum. Spend the other ninety percent of your time building better habits to lose fat and keep it off.

The Law of Imperfect Progress
No diet is perfect. Intermittent fasting. Paleo. Atkins. Mediterranean. South Beach. Ketogenic. But they can all work by restricting choices, so you eat fewer calories, more protein, and more vegetables. That is it.

There is no perfect diet. Do not fall in love with the fancy marketing methods of any diet. Focus on core principles instead. Eat less, move more, crush vegetables, and eat a high protein diet.

The Law of Metabolic Compensation
This law illustrates the adaptive and reactive nature of metabolism. The metabolism is constantly seeking balance or homeostasis. As a result, when you push on the metabolism in any direction, it will push back against you.

This is much like a tug-o-war against an unbeatable opponent. The only way to win such a game is to let go of the rope so the other team goes tumbling helplessly to the ground.

You can do this with your metabolism by learning to play a different type of game than "eat less, exercise more." Most people use this simplistic mantra, and therefore view the metabolism as a calculator. They believe it has a linear, predictable, and stable function. All that's necessary is to punch in the right numbers and weight loss utopia is achieved. Of course, this isn't true in practice.

The Law of Flexible Dieting
Adopt a flexible dieting approach and forgive yourself for diet slip-ups. My definition of flexible dieting is eating right 80% of the time, then allowing yourself the occasional cheat meal before getting back on your diet. **Fitness should improve your life, not consume it.** When you slip up, have a short memory. Forgive yourself. Forgive and make the next best decision. The stricter you are with hitting your diet 100% perfect 100% of the time the more likely you'll go insane, develop a case of the "fuck-its" and quit.

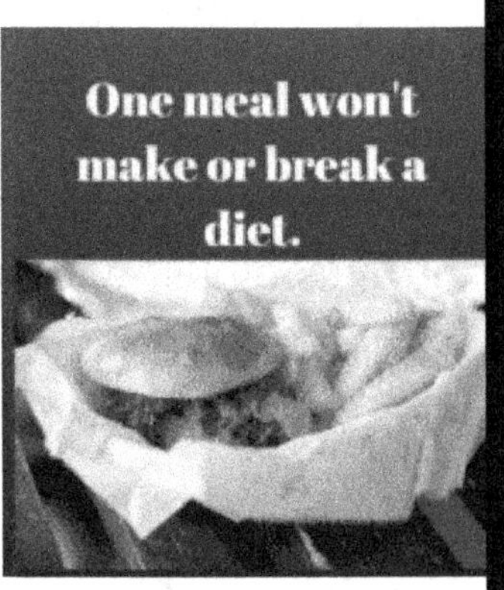

One meal won't ruin a diet and one Oreo doesn't need to be a whole carton of Oreos. A life obsessed with diet and body composition isn't a life at all. Make the best decisions most of the time, forgive yourself for the slip-up, and get back on track.

The Law of Strength Training
The purpose of lifting weights is to build strength and muscle. The role of weight training in a diet is to preserve the strength and muscle you already have. You'll maintain anabolic hormone levels like testosterone and growth hormone, both of which support higher lean muscle mass and less fat mass.

This results in faster fat loss and reveals a strong, lean, and aesthetic body…not the dreaded skinny fat look from crummy training during a diet.

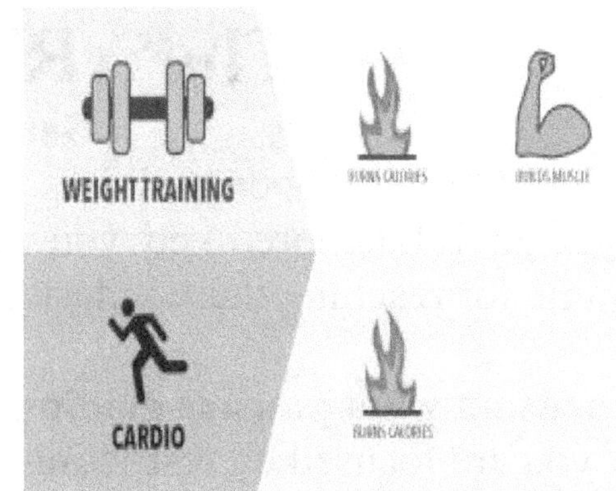

Lift heavy at least once per week if you want to stay strong and muscular during a fat loss diet.

Upper Body: Overhead press, chin-up, bench press, dip, row
Lower Body: Clean, squat, deadlift, lunge

Start with a moderate load and increase weight by 5-10% each set, aiming to reach your heaviest set in 4-6 sets. Ramping sets works better to avoid excess fatigue in your already depleted state.

___

The Law of Singular Focus
You can get stronger, lose fat, and build muscle…but pick one at a time.

This is because at any given moment your body is either anabolic (building, such as building muscle or accumulating fat mass) or catabolic (breaking down fat, muscle, or carbohydrates for energy). This means at any given moment you're either losing fat or gaining muscle…but not both. So, this would lead you to believe you can't build muscle and lose fat at the same time, right?
You can. While your body can only build or breakdown fuel at one time, it can switch between phases of being anabolic and catabolic throughout the day. For most people chasing simultaneous fat loss and muscle building it is the first-class ticket to spin your wheels for weeks and months, hopping from program to program and diet to diet.

Go all in with one goal, make it happen, then switch gears.

Execute the Basics
Most people want to lose fat, get healthy, and look better naked. Fewer educate themselves on what works. After that, less than 10% of people are willing to do what it takes. Which one are you?

INSTEAD OF.....	TRY THINKING....
I'm not good at this	What am I missing?
I give up	I'll use a different strategy
It's good enough	Is this really my best work?
I can't make this any better	I can always improve
This is too hard	This may take some time
I made a mistake	Mistakes help me to learn
I just can't do this	I am going to train my brain
I'll never be that smart	I will learn how to do this
Plan A didn't work	There's always Plan B
My friend can do it	I will learn from them

The ART of effective Goal setting

Get Specific and avoid "vague" goals.

Weight loss is a poor goal. It is too general and lacks focus. The more specific you are with your goals the more likely you will be to reach them. How much weight loss? What is your time frame for reaching these milestones? What are you willing to do to achieve these results?

Focus on what you are gaining, not on what you are giving up.

If you are focused on restricting items from your life and view improving fitness levels/exercise as a chore, or you are focused on eliminating foods from your life - how long do you think you will have the willpower to hold out? A better strategy is to list out all the things you will gain by making changes to your habits. Improved energy and self-confidence would most likely happen first. Self-pride and the ability to stick with your goals and plans would follow.

Get into the process and out of the outcome.

Change takes time. Be patient. No one makes one decision and then magically changes. Everyone makes mistakes and takes missteps. Understand that a mistake is not the end. Get right back on track and get going. Improved fitness and reduced weight of any substantial sum is most likely a 12-18-month process. There will be plateaus and setbacks. How you plan for and deal with these setbacks will make all the difference in your success. You WILL NOT experience smooth sailing. And, if you do, you will not maintain it for long.

Focus on your schedule. If you schedule it, you will do it.

For many people sticking to a schedule is difficult. The habit of procrastination sets in, and what I refer to as "The Tomorrow Syndrome," becomes a rally cry. If you will always start tomorrow and justify your lack of commitment to your health and goals, you will never reach the goals that you set. Schedule your exercise and stick to your schedule. Make your fitness a non-negotiable priority. If you do not- you will not achieve the desired results.

Avoid "All or None" thinking.

Focus on progress, not perfection. If you are moving more than you have been before and eating better than you have then you are making progress! Congratulate yourself. You are doing great.

The fastest or the best?

We do not want the *fastest* way to lose weight. We want the *best* way. The best way makes us healthier, not just smaller. The best way makes us stronger, not weaker. The best way builds sustainable habits that can become a lifestyle. The best way is safe and supports heart health, brain health, and longevity. The best way gets the body fat down and the muscle mass up. The best way is one friends and the whole family can follow and enjoy together. The best way teaches us to skip the quick fix and instead invest some challenging work and discipline today for a rewarding return down the road. The best way is medicine for body and mind. The fastest way isn't the best way, and the best way isn't the fastest.

PLAY-span vs LIFEspan

Every man dies. Not every man truly lives! – William Wallace - Braveheart

Play-Span™ is a concept create by Neal Spruce. With it, Neal separates how long we live vs how long we are disease free and ultimately, how long we have the vitality and ability to do that which we love. In this discussion, I will take the concept and add measureables for Health-Span and Play-Span.

First, his definitions -

Life-Span - How long you live.

Health-Span - How long you're healthy: functional & disease-free period of life.

Play-Span™ - How long you're physically/mentally able to do activities important to you.

Put into action, the differentiation between health and play begin to take shape. You can remain relatively healthy but not able to enjoy play and vice versa. In our modern society, we are more likely to see someone lose their ability to play well before they lose their health. Obviously, this is not the case in all circumstances, however, it is more likely due to increased sedentary living and more frequent high-calorie, low-nutrition food choices repeated over years.

I think it is important to note that I am not passing judgement on anyone's individual choices. On the contrary, I believe fully that if you take responsibility for the choices and the repercussion(s) of your choice, no one should tell you what is best for you. This discussion, more so, is about how to measure and qualify your health-span and your play-span. It is for the people striving for vitality.

As you will see, Play-Span has little to do with age and much to do with ageing.

Goal – Honest assessment of your current abilities and habits.

Outcome – Create a short-term and long-term plan that enables you to do what you love for as long as your health-span and lifespan allow.

"Your lifestyle determines your death style: - James Hetfield – Metallica

James makes a great point here. Is he talking about stepping off a curb and getting hit by a car? If you are reckless and staring at your phone while walking near traffic, maybe. More likely (and for our purposes) he is speaking about the controllable factors such as exercising, eating right sleeping enough, avoid smoking (and now vaping too) and other such factors discussed below.

The reason lifestyle is so important is because how you live determines your choices and these choices decide how healthy you are and whether you're on the road to weight loss, fitness and sustained health. So, what is a healthy lifestyle? Where do you fall on the healthy lifestyle continuum?

My **PLAYSPAN markers** for movement that I use as a checklist -

1) Can you squat down with your butt between your shoes on demand?
2) Can you touch your toes?
3) Can you reach your arms straight above your head (airplane luggage bin, tall shelf)?
4) Can you put your socks on while standing up or alternately, can you stand on 1 leg for 30 seconds?
5) Can you drive your car in reverse while turning around to see where you are going (not using a backup camera)?
6) Can you sleep using one pillow for your head?
7) Can you walk a mile at a brisk pace without stopping?
8) Can you "freely" get in and out of your car?
9) Can you stand up from a chair without using upper-body help?
10) Can you get to the ground and back up to standing without using your arms?
11) Can you climb and descend a flight of stairs without pain?

Basically, can you do the motions/movements that are simple? Age-related breakdown is normal. Accelerated ageing is a choice.

Health-Span markers – (important note – this section is NOT healthcare advice; it is simply a group of questions to increase awareness).

1) Are you currently at what is considered a healthy weight?
2) Are you currently within acceptable standards of bodyfat?
3) Is your blood pressure considered healthy?
4) What is your resting heart rate?
5) How many medications are you currently taking?
6) Do you drink at least ½ of your Bodyweight in ounces of water daily?
7) Do you sleep 6-8 hours per night?
8) Do you have healthy stress management techniques?
9) Do you have healthy and supportive relationships?

Quantify then Modify

This questionnaire will allow you to quantify your habits, both good and not so good, allowing you an honest opportunity
Diving into the specifics - First, figure out how much time you spend doing the following:

Hours per Day	Hours Per Week	
		Sitting at a desk
		Sitting in a car
		Sitting in front of a TV
		Sitting in front of a computer
		Eating out at restaurants
		Drinking alcohol
		Eating fast food or junk foods
		Staying up late/not getting enough sleep

Now, how much time do you spend?

Hours per Day	Hours Per Week	
		Being active in general
		Doing cardio exercise
		Strength training with challenging weights
		Preparing your own healthy meals and snacks
		Reading food labels
		Tracking your calories
		Sleeping
		Dealing with stress in a healthy way

If you spend more time doing the things in the first list than the second, it's time to reevaluate your priorities and decide what you really want for yourself. Living healthy means spending time and energy on your body--moving it around and paying attention to what you put into it. Staying in an unhealthy lifestyle means you can avoid expending energy, time and effort...but at what cost?

 Innovation Fitness Solutions – Achievers Success Guide

Choosing Health and Fitness for High Performance Living

As humans, we like habits and routines, so much that we often keep doing the same things even when we know they are not good for us. Changing bad habits takes time and effort and, for a healthy lifestyle, you may be changing a variety of things like:

What time you get up each morning?

What time you go to bed each night?

How you spend your free time?

How you spend your money?

How you shop, cook and eat?

How much TV you watch?

What you do with your family and friends?

How much time do you spend planning your week?

Current:	New Habit:

Eating Habits Assessment
Take stock of your environment and your thought process prior to and during eating times. Create the proper environment and utilize the correct tools for consistent changes.
1. **Your Current eating habits.**
   - Do you eat at desk?
   - Where and how do you eat most of your meals?
   - What do you eat during these times?
   - How will this be compatible with your new food choices?

2. **Are you prepared to eat differently than your friends at social functions?**
   - Eating often accompanies many social gatherings. How do your friends eat?
   - Do they consume foods that you know will not be compatible with your lifestyle?
   - How will you address this?

3. **Are you prepared to change your home environment?**
   - Does your home environment work with your new plans? You may have chosen to eat mindfully and leisurely. The trouble is your home is utterly chaotic, noisy, and messy, with barely a place to sit down, let alone have a large, pleasant space to indulge in your new meals.
   - What will you do to change this?

 Innovation Fitness Solutions – Achievers Success Guide

4. How do your current habits fit?
- What if your leisure activities always involve eating junk food?
- What happens if you start a diet that completely rules out junk food?
- What will you do? Change your habits? Find a different comfort food?

5. What about eating away from home?
- Do you eat at restaurants a lot?
- Which restaurants do you go to?
- Will they fit with your new style of eating?
- Are you prepared to leave food on your plate if their portions are too big?

6. Is your kitchen set-up properly?
- Look around your kitchen.
- Do you have enough fridge/freezer space?
- Do you have proper cookware?
- Do you have enough containers? Enough time?

7. Are you being totally honest with yourself?
- You read about a new diet in a magazine, and it requires eating a lot more vegetables. On the surface you are busting to lose "10 pounds in 2 weeks", but deep down you know you cannot stand vegetables. Which part of you will win out in the end?
- Why do you hate veggies? Are you prepared to cook more, or learn different ways of cooking them?

8. Can you accept the things you cannot change?
- You cannot change the way other people act and the way they speak - "oh, so you're on another health kick, again are you?" But you can choose ahead of time how you will respond inwardly and outwardly.

9. Will you continue monitoring yourself objectively?
- Many people reach their ideal weight, and then let old habits creep back in. However, there are a few warning systems in place. One is the waistband in your pants. Will you choose to conveniently ignore it if it gets tighter? Or will you be objective?

10. How will the lifestyle of family and friends affect your health/weight loss efforts?
- If your entire world is filled with people who are couch potatoes, how do you plan to work against this culture?
- Will they influence you to be more active or more sedentary?

My hope is that by performing this simple assessment, you can glean insight into your lifestyle that may be ignored and begin to create a plan for a lifestyle that allows you to maximize your play-span.

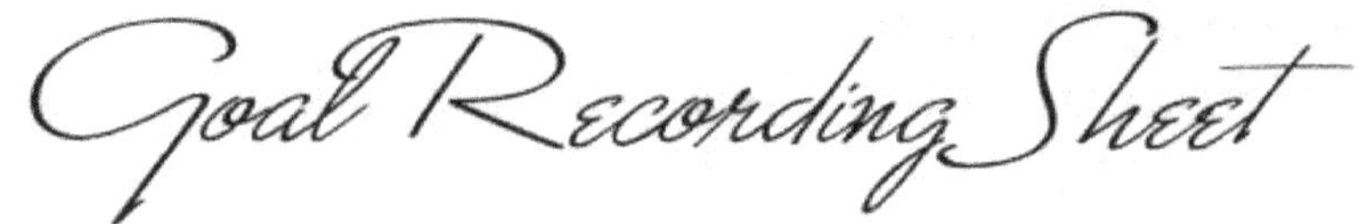

Long Range Goal: ____

   I. Short Range Goal: ______________________________________

       A. Step 1: ______________________________________

       B. Step 2: ______________________________________

       C. Step 3: ______________________________________

   II. Short Range Goal: ______________________________________

       A. Step 1: ______________________________________

       B. Step 2: ______________________________________

       C. Step 3: ______________________________________

   III. Short Range Goal: ______________________________________

       A. Step 1: ______________________________________

       B. Step 2: ______________________________________

       C. Step 3: ______________________________________

   IV. Short Range Goal: ______________________________________

       A. Step 1: ______________________________________

       B. Step 2: ______________________________________

       C. Step 3: ______________________________________

Mantras to keep you mentally strong

While it is often easy to be mentally strong when life is going well, your true strength becomes apparent through adversity. The loss of a loved one, a health problem, relationship issues, and financial troubles are just a few of the hardships most people face at one time or another. The way you think about life's inevitable obstacles affects your ability to cope with tough times. Developing a productive inner dialogue is one of the most productive ways mentally strong people build mental muscle. Repeating positive, yet realistic affirmations can drown out the negative thoughts that can hold you back. Here are nine things to remember when you are going through tough times.

1. I have what I need to get through this.
Thinking things like "I can't do this" or "This isn't fair" will cause you to feel defeated. Rather than insist you need more, remember what you already have. If you have made it this far in life, you clearly have some skills, tools, and resources already in place.

2. Living according to my values is what really matters.
There are going to be people who will not like you and times when people will disagree with the decisions you make. But your job is not to please everyone. Be brave enough to live according to your values, even when that means making unpopular decisions.

3. Failure is part of the road to success.
Failure is not fun but beating yourself up over it will not help. Each time you fall, it serves as proof you're pushing yourself to new limits. Remember that each failure is an opportunity to grow stronger and become better.

4. All I can do is my best.
Demanding perfection from yourself will do more harm than good. Whether you are interviewing for a job that you really need, or you've got one last shot to try for that promotion, insisting there's no room for error will skyrocket your anxiety. A little self-compassion will help you perform at your peak.

5. Five years from now this won't matter as much as I think it will.
Keep temporary problems in perspective by reminding yourself that the emotional pain, anxiety, or turmoil won't last forever. Many of today's crucial decisions and major worries won't matter that much a few years down the road.

6. I'm stronger than I think.
A serious health problem or the loss of a loved one can be very difficult to handle. But catastrophic predictions like "I'll never recover from this" or "I won't ever be happy again" will only drag you down. Adversity often reveals hidden inner strength you never knew you had.

7. I can handle feeling uncomfortable.
It can be tempting to stay inside your comfort zone but getting through tough times often requires you to do something different. Although emotions like fear, embarrassment, and disappointment are uncomfortable, they will not kill you. Be willing to face those emotions head on and you will gain confidence in your ability to cope with discomfort.

8. I am in control of how I think, feel, and behave.
Blaming other people for what is going on in your life will not help your situation. Acknowledging that you are in control of how you think, feel, and behave can empower you to either make the best of your circumstances, or create positive changes in your life.

9. I have been knocked down before and I can get back up again.
Look back at the times you have persevered before. Recalling your fortitude in dealing with past struggles can help you summon the strength to deal with current problems.

Giving yourself positive affirmations alone will not necessarily change your life, but healthy self-talk will help you feel better and inspire you to behave more productively, which is key to getting through tough times.

Becoming aware of what, when, how and why you eat can help to lose weight

Slow down - Remember to be mindful about your food choices and eating habits.

Be patient with yourself - Changing behaviors is a long process, but it is also long-lasting. Results are not and will never be linear. Expect lots of ups and downs.

Expect to slip up - Don't even entertain the idea of perfection. If there were no mistakes, there'd be nothing to learn from. If you "blow it today, make a plan for tomorrow that includes solutions to the difficulties.

Determine your overeating cues - If you're overeating often - you're just putting a band-aid on a gaping wound. Try to determine the root cause of what's eating you by following the recommendations above.

Motivation follows action - That is, getting motivated to change your eating patterns isn't going to hit you someday. You must act first. When you see results, you will be motivated to continue.

You can do this! Believe in yourself today!

HONESTY COVENANT

Do you want to know why people are forever challenged to achieve their goals? An HONESTY COVENANT is essential to continued progress. If you choose these "loopholes", even occasionally, then these choices accumulate.

What are you doing consistently to DESERVE attaining your goals? I am not talking about being a good person etc... I am talking about the consistent actions to bring progress.

*Which of these is you? *

1. **False choice loophole** - "I can't do this, because I'm so busy doing that"

2. **Moral licensing loophole** - "I've been so good, it's okay for me to do this"

3. **Tomorrow loophole** - "It's okay to skip today, because I'm going to do this tomorrow"

4. **Lack of control loophole** - "I can't help myself"

5. **Planning to fail loophole, formerly known as the "Apparently irrelevant decision loophole"** - "I'll just check my email quickly before I go to the gym…oops, I don't have time to go to the gym, after all."

6. **"This doesn't count" loophole** – "I'm on vacation", "I'm sick", "It's the weekend"

7. **Questionable assumption loophole** - "It's not a proper dinner without wine; This is taking too long, I should be done already; I can't start working until my office is clean; I'm too busy to take the stairs. It's faster to wait in this long elevator line; The label says it's healthy."

8. **Concern for others loophole** - "I can't do this because it might make other people uncomfortable"

9. **Fake self-actualization loophole** – "You only live once! Embrace the moment!"

10. **One-coin loophole** – "What difference does it make if I break my habit this one time?"

11. **Rebellion loophole** - To hell with this! I am going to eat a doughnut today!

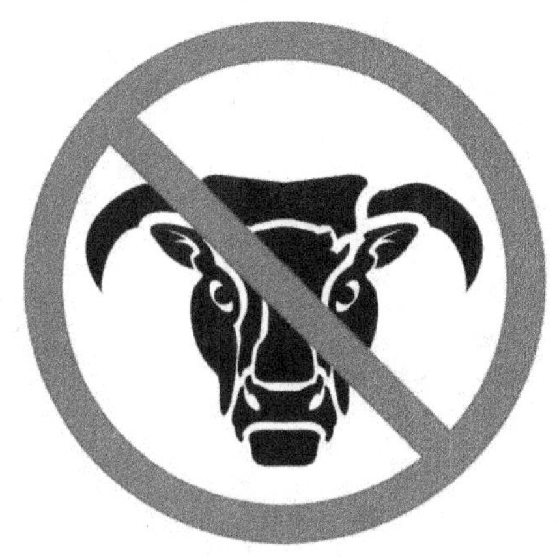

Overcoming the Fear of Failure

One of the biggest hindrances to productivity and success is fear. Whether the issue is weight loss, learning a new skill, making a career move or any number of other activities, we are most paralyzed by fear of failure. But failure is part of our lives; it is not going to go away. The best way to deal with a fear of failure is to change our mindset about it, so that we can move beyond inactivity and start making remarkable things happen in our lives.

Change your mindset.

There is a sure way to avoid failure, and that is to never attempt anything. But never attempting anything is not success either; in fact, it is to barely exist at all. Anyone who takes action and pursues anything is going to fail, but successful people see their failure as steps in the learning process. Combating fear of failure demands that you expect failure to show up at some point, because there is no way to avoid it. This does not mean that you do not also expect success. It simply means that you dive in with the full understanding that most successes have a track record of bumps and stumbles. The truly successful person realizes that she may fall, but when she falls she will get right back up again, take stock of what she has learned and then move forward again. Use the following strategy to tackle your fear of failure and start making some epic changes in your life:

1. Visualize the failure.

So, what if you do fail? What will that look like? How will you react? What will your next move be? Considering the worst-case scenario and how you will deal with it helps you make friends with the possibility of failure and takes away the uncertainty. Recognizing and embracing the possibility of failure diffuses its power to paralyze you. When you have a plan, the road looks much safer.

2. Start.

The first step is the hardest, but after you take that first action step, you will have momentum that will keep propelling you forward. What is the first thing you need to do to start the process of your venture? Do you need to make a phone call? Write a to-do list? Write a business proposal? Pick the first, small action you need to take and just do it.

Success seldom comes without failure. Embrace it and go forward from here.

THE SPECTRUM OF SUCCESS

Keeping a positive attitude and rid yourself of those negative thoughts forever.

First: Every morning when you wake up, say something positive about yourself and your commitment to live a healthier lifestyle. For example: "I like myself and I'm committed to a healthier lifestyle."

Next: After your workouts, always have a positive attitude about the workout and the way you are feeling at that moment. Your endorphins will be peaking, and this will help to promote a positive outlook.

Then: Praise yourself for the demanding work and commitment you made to complete your routine. Even if it was not the best workout you have ever had, it was still a workout. "Something is better than nothing" is the attitude you need to have.

Expand: Spread your positive energy to the rest of the world. Compliment at least one person daily. The compliment can be about someone's shoes, tie, smile, eyes, or something that just pops out at you about that person. When you do this, more positive energy will come into your life. This is called the Law of Giving and Receiving. If you put positive energy out, it will come back to you. If you put negative energy out, it will also come back to you.

Last: Before you go to bed, say something positive about yourself and reaffirm your commitment to live a healthier lifestyle. As you begin to understand your reasons for negative self-talk, you will find yourself recognizing it more and more quickly when it occurs. Eventually, as you practice, you will be able to recognize and stop negative self-talk before it interferes with your decisions.

It is especially important to practice positive thinking and to remind yourself that you are a worthwhile person. Consistently acknowledge that you are making positive changes to improve your health. You should be proud of yourself. Visualize yourself as capable, happy, and confident. These positive feelings will help the process of change.

Getting over Failures and moving forward.

- What is past is all said and done. What remains to be seen is what I can bring to my present and future.
- Better for me to concentrate on what I am doing today rather than on what I did or did not do before. What I do today will shape my tomorrows. The past is not going to get any better!
- Poor decisions made in the past do not have to be repeated in the present.
- Because something happened once does not mean that it must continue to happen.
- No matter how bad any event was I do not have to allow it to continue to have a negative influence on my life. I cannot rewrite history and change what has already happened.

- Feeling sorry for myself, angry toward others, guilty, or ashamed for getting the short end of the stick in the past will only continue to keep me from achieving happiness in the present and future.
- What I tell myself today is much more important than what others have told me in the past.
- My experiences do not represent *me.* Rather, they represent *things I have experienced;* they do not make me into a better or worse person and do not determine my future success.

Maintaining Your Strong Mind

1. **Success comes first in the mind,** so visualize yourself accomplishing your goals.
2. Remember, you are the only person who can hold you back.
3. **Forgive yourself** and love yourself despite past failures.
4. Decide what is important in your life and focus on that.
5. **Conquer each negative thought the moment it enters your mind** when it is weakest.
6. Give up the idea that things will not go right unless you worry about them.
7. If you bring the body of your dreams to the point of resolve, you will soon be living in it.
8. Look towards your future, **if you believe the best is yet to come then it will be.**
9. You become what you think about most.
10. The margin between success and failure is exceedingly small and easily bridged by determination.
11. Start your day by accomplishing your hardest task first.
12. **Set small attainable goals,** rather than one monumental goal.
13. Convince yourself that exercise is fun, and it will be.
14. Know your big reason 'why'.
15. **Create a motivating play list of songs** to use as the soundtrack to your workout sessions.
16. Every decision either leads you closer toward achieving your goal, or farther from it.
17. If you think you are a fat person, then you will stay fat. **If you think you are fit, then you soon will be.**
18. Once you have set your goal, your attitude either pushes you toward accomplishment or failure.
19. If you do not know exactly where you want to go, you will likely end up someplace else.
20. You can have the body of your dreams, but **first you must give up the belief that you cannot.**
21. You can only have two things in life: excuses or results – choose the latter.

Read these 21 Tips over again, identify where YOU need more help and work at it.

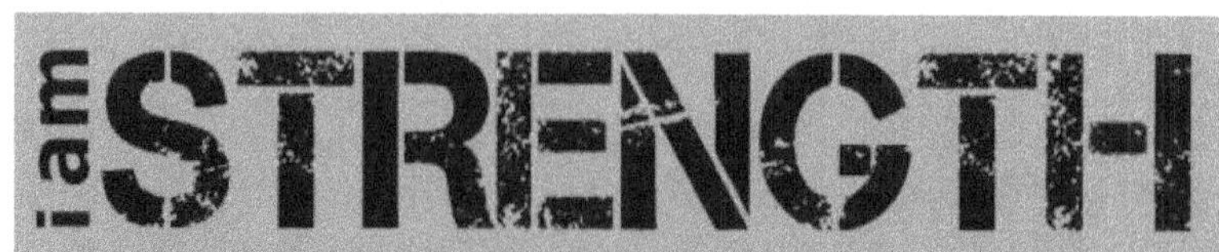

The Stages of Transformation

Having identifiable and realistic expectations is a crucial step to remain consistent, offset setbacks and achieve lasting results. The **Stages of Transformation** explains the physical and mental process we often experience. The confusion of what, how and why things occur (or do not) is normal, and frustration can dampen motivation while sapping patience. The explanations are not intended to be linear, nor is it the process that everyone will experience. It is an outline of the average experiences of decades of client feedback. Keep in mind that with life transformation, you are tackling many processes at once, and your ability to be successful with some while struggling with others is normal.

Stage 1 – Metabolic Recovery
Your first 30-60 days

During this initial period, your motivation is exceedingly high and so, too, are your expectations. You have made the ultimate decision to change your weight and your life and you expect impressive results immediately. Your expectations, your actions and your outcomes will be at odds. A successful paradigm shift is necessary for you to find the long-term success you desire. This period is mainly spent on learning new tools and skills to ensure you understand how your body functions and reacts to different foods and stimuli. This time will also be spent correcting a few key nutritional and lifestyle imbalances, learning to deal with minor setbacks and learning proper goal setting techniques.

- Metabolic Recovery is initiated by ending yo-yo dieting.
- Temporary weight fluctuations from hormonal balance, rehydrating the body, strength increases and function from overcoming sarcopenia (adult muscle loss) and years of yo-yo dieting.
- Better food choices and awareness of decisions and choices in life will improve your understanding of the damage from years of chronic, failed dieting.
- You will experience increased energy and focus.
- You will feel steady (sometimes surprising) strength increases.
- At times, you will experience increased confusion and frustration.
  - Your beliefs about yourself and weight loss in general are at odds with your current actions and traditions. You are doing something different than what you have typically done to get "results". You are frustrated that the scale has not dropped 10 lbs. and that you are not at your "goal" yet.
  - Overall feeling: "Why is this taking so long? But I feel so much better and exercise is not nearly as "bad" as I thought." Exercising is viewed as somewhat enjoyable but for the most part is still a chore.
  - Often, you feel like giving up, that this is "too hard" and/or that you want to quit and try something else, but if you are honest with yourself and know that the other methods you have tried in the past have failed you., you learn to gain mental and emotional strength from your positive support group. Not to mention, you remain open to the coaching from the IFS Coaches and to the support of others.

- Your relationship with food has gone from mindlessness (eating for taste and convenience and stemming from boredom and emotionally driven) to now being too strict. Basically, you were eating following no rules; now you have created too many rules.

Stage 2 - Improved Fitness
Days 45 – 90

You are gaining Lean Body Mass, boosting energy, feeling much more energetic, sleeping better, and noticing changes in how your clothes fit, how your body feels and the additional abilities you now have. This is great!

- You continue to get stronger and feel fit.
- Typically, there still is minimal (if any) weight loss but you are noticing that your clothes are fitting differently and seeing changes in the mirror. This is due to eating better, drinking more water, strength training and the consistency of your actions.

You are also beginning to understand the methods that you are employing, and you are feeling and seeing results even though you still may be confused because the scale has not moved how you though that it should.

- You now have ownership over the fact that you have abandoned 'Instant Gratification' and are utilizing long-term success methods to match your long-term goals.
- Feeling decreased stress. "Small stuff" is not bothering you nearly as much and you are beginning to feel confident instead of confused.
- Improved sleep and generally, more satisfaction from life.
- Overall feeling – "This is beginning to make sense."
- Your relationship with food is improving, moving from having too many rules to understanding the true meaning of balanced eating for nutrition, satiety, satisfaction and performance.
- Exercise is now enjoyable and rewarding rather than viewed as a punishment.

Stage 3 - Transformation
Month 4 to 1 year

You have built a foundation of quality, health and performance enhancing habits. You are working out consistently, your strength levels have increased, and you can perform more work. Your nutrition is continually improving, and your energy levels are high.

The 4 methods of change			
START a completely new action	STOP doing something entirely	Do MORE of something	Do LESS of something

- NOW you begin to experience steady weight loss.
- You have gained LBM and this event has reached its maintenance level.
- You are maintaining a calorie deficit and making better, healthier choices to allow Fat Loss to continue.
- New habits have taken effect and you continue to gain strength physically and mentally.
- Mentally, you are moving from the cry of "Weight Loss" to understanding what it takes to reach your ACTUAL transformation goals.

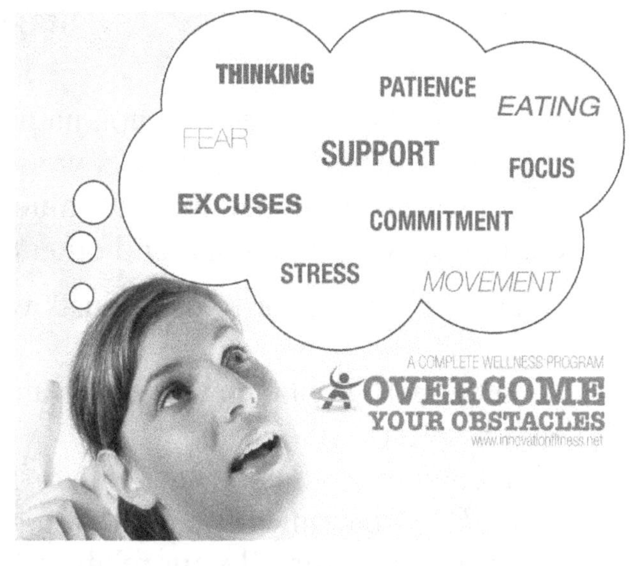

- You have complete ownership of your responsibility to take care of yourself.
- You no longer stress about "small stuff", you understand your long-term goals and health vision and have powerful self-talk which allows you to make choices instead of succumbing to reactions.
- Near the end of this year you begin to consider different goals.
    - Conflicting thoughts range from desiring more weight loss or "forcing" more weight loss to being confused about what to do next.
    - You have become accustomed to attempting to lose weight for years (employing different methods) and now that you are well on your way, you begin to focus on different goals for your life but are anchored in what you have always known.

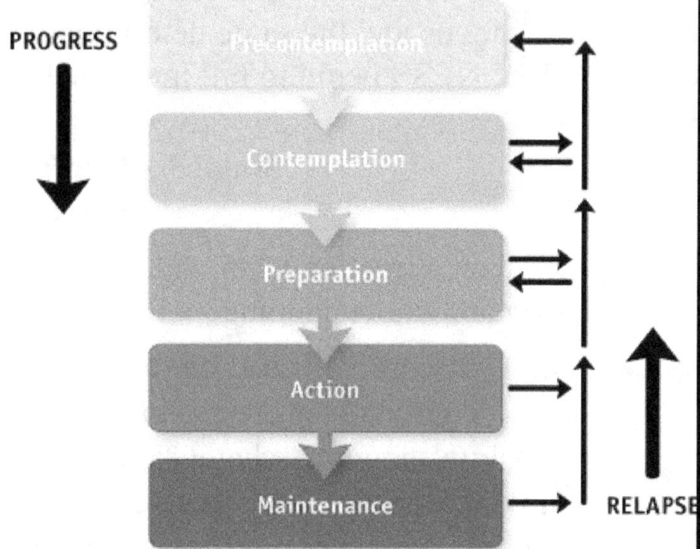

Your relationship with food has evolved from no rules to too many rules to where you are now "Structured Flexibility". You understand the needs of your body, what and how to feed it and are just as concerned with optimal performance as you are with appearance. Your view of fitness is healthy. You partake in regular, structured fitness training and live an active lifestyle. You enjoy the outdoors and get the IFSism – Flowers, Birds & Trees. You have enhanced focus and consistently look for ways to challenge yourself mentally and physically. You fully understand what you are doing and why you are doing it. Doubt and confusion are being replaced with confidence. You continue to learn new strategies and tools to aid in your understanding of nutrition, fitness, and mindset.

 Innovation Fitness Solutions – Achievers Success Guide

Stage 4 – Wellness
1 year to 2 years

Through Personal Growth efforts you naturally transition to focusing on various aspects of "growing your life". Weight loss is now viewed as a side effect of your better habits and your decision-making is grounded in your values and your long-term needs. As with any evolution, your relationships with yourself and others have changed significantly.

- Wellness takes priority over "just" weight loss and you begin searching for more out of life.
- You begin to create new interests and/or hobbies or rekindle your love for things you had given up on.
- You challenge yourself to create different and more personal, meaningful goals.
- Your focus becomes one of creating and maintaining a fantastic relationship with yourself, allowing all your relationships that you choose to be in to flourish.
- Life slows down for you. You are focused on solution-based thinking instead of the challenges and issues. Your decisions are based on your core values and this allows you to act much quicker without deliberation.
- You are at (or awfully close to) a healthy weight and living a healthy, fit lifestyle.
- You are active in recreation and relationships.
- With focus and the same determination that it took to "learn" weight loss, all aspects of WELLNESS begin to fall into place for you.

Stage 5 – Life Transformation - "Being"
The Rest of Your Life

You operate on a trusting level with yourself. Doubt has been replaced by confidence, compassion and understanding.

- You own your values and priorities.
  - Your choices are driven from these.
- Life slows down to whatever speed you are comfortable with and you experience true enjoyment, peace, and success.
- Thinking and inner conflict is replaced by "Being".

Congratulations! You have achieved your true goals and intentions.

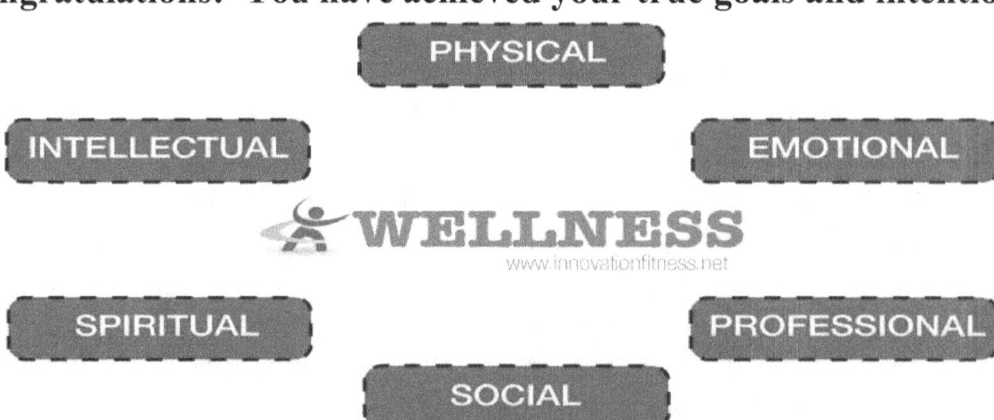

WEIGHT CONTROL BASICS

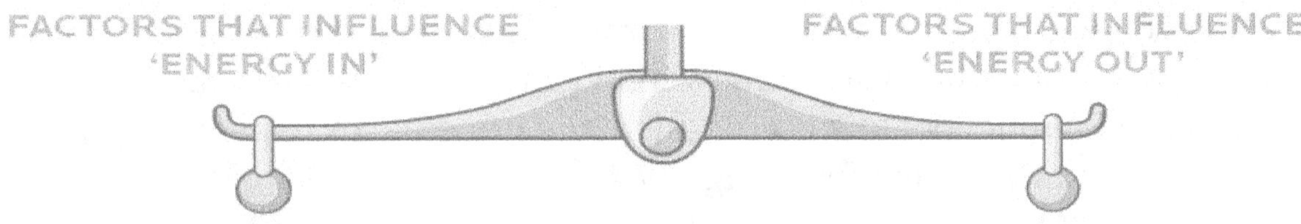

APPETITE
Influenced by hormones that regulate appetite and satiety

ENERGY BURNED AT REST
Influenced by body size, hormonal status, dieting history, genetic factors, health status, sleep quality, age

FOOD CONSUMED
Influenced by availability, palatability, energy density, sleep quality, education, socioeconomic status, culture

ENERGY BURNED THROUGH EXERCISE
Influenced by exercise ability, intensity, duration, frequency, type, environment, as well as hormonal status and sleep quality

CALORIES ABSORBED
Influenced by macronutrient intake, food prep, age, personal microbiome, health status, energy status

ENERGY BURNED BY NON-EXERCISE ACTIVITY
Influenced by health status, energy status, stress levels, hormonal status, occupation, leisure activities, genetic factors

PSYCHOLOGICAL FACTORS
Influenced by stress levels, mindset, perceived control, self-esteem, sleep quality

ENERGY BURNED BY METABOLIZING FOOD
Influenced by macronutrient makeup and how processed the food is

This isn't a comprehensive list of factors, but rather a snapshot of the most common ones. It's important to know that elements on both sides of the scale are influenced by: each other, hormones (e.g. leptin, thyroid), sleep, stress, medical conditions, pharmaceuticals, and more. This means none of these things invalidate CICO. Rather, they influence how many calories we absorb and how many we burn. And this is what leads to weight gain or loss.

How and why do we gain weight?

Ultimately, your weight is determined by the calories you take in and the calories you burn daily. If you are like most adults, you have been taking in more calories than you burn, and you have excess body fat that you would like to get rid of. If you are not like most adults, consider yourself warned, as experts predict that 9 out of 10 people will become overweight or obese at some point in their lifetime. This underscores the importance of consistently balancing the calories you take in with the right amount of activity, especially since most people gain weight slowly and steadily without really noticing it. Years of misjudging your intake by just a few calories at a time will end up sabotaging your weight. For example, if you gain the average amount of one pound per year, this means you are off by only 10 calories each day. After 20 to 30 years, you will end up 20 to 30 pounds' overweight. To help you avoid this, here are common ways people underestimate the calories they take in and unknowingly eat more than they realize.

So why have most adults become overweight or obese in recent decades? We have taken in more fuel (calories) than the body burns mostly because of lifestyle changes. Think about it, manual labor is now performed by machines and computers, very few calories are burned during our daily routine because work, transportation, recreation, and entertainment are mostly sedentary. People eat out more frequently and enticing food is offered everywhere in copious quantities, day, or night. Because we (humans) have a natural tendency to preserve energy and eat even when we are not hungry, modern lifestyle easily leads to unburned fuel and unwanted weight gain.

There are many reasons why this caloric imbalance occurs, however, fundamentally, you only gain weight when you have an energy (calorie) surplus. Learning to control this surplus through a myriad of methods will aid you in stopping weight gain and allow for a caloric deficit. Vitally important and repeated throughout this book will be the principle of maintaining your muscle tissue while focusing on fat loss, not just weight loss.

The scale never lies long-term.

On any given day, the scale can deceive you and your true progress will not be accurately reflected by your weight. This is because body weight can fluctuate daily due to the amount of fluid we retain (see Bodyweight Range). Foods high in sodium, menstrual cycles, certain medications, and bowel movements can increase fluid retention and skew your weight. Therefore, I suggest that you gain a proper perspective in using the scale as a tool in weight maintenance. Daily weighing (or more often) generally leads to consistent disappointment due to unrealistic expectations. Committing to weighing yourself only once per week can help keep your mindset focused on the long-term happening in your calorie intake.

Over time the scale does tell the whole story. If your weight creeps up after two or three weeks, you have been eating more calories than you are burning. The opposite is also true – if your weight decreases after two to three weeks, you have been eating fewer calories than you are burning. A steady weight indicates the calories you are burning, and consuming are equal.

Weight gain typically happens slowly…
The average yearly weight gain among adults is one to
three pounds. This means most people are off by only
20 to 30 calories a day. Minor changes such as
skipping those last few bites or taking 200-300 extra
steps per day will keep you trim and away from weight
loss diets. But keep in mind as you get older, you are
likely to burn fewer calories because your daily routine
and metabolism changes. Because of this, you will

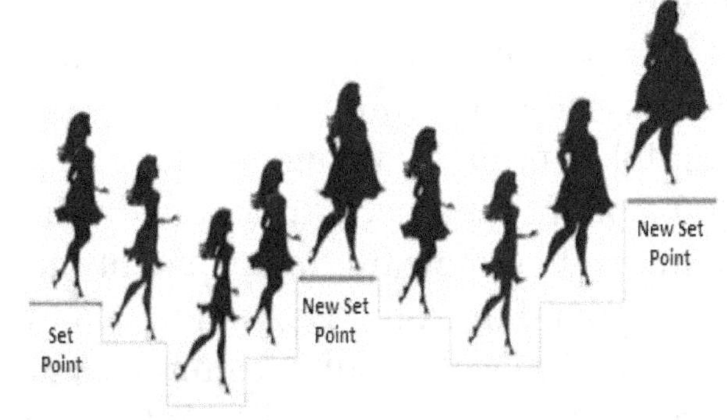

have to become aware of the calories you take in and how much, or how little, you move. To
keep your weight in check, you will need to get on the scale or measure your waistline more
than once a year. I strongly urge you to self-weigh once per week to keep undesired weight gain
in check.

How much do we *really* eat?
Let's say you do know how many calories to eat to manage your weight. The next question is -
do you accurately judge how much food you eat? Not according to research. When people are
asked to record how much they consume, they consistently underestimate. Overweight and
obese women tend to underestimate more than other people, and it worsens as body mass index
(BMI) goes up. That is, the higher the BMI, the fewer calories people report eating. Meal size
also affects how accurate we are. The larger the meal, the more we misjudge how much we eat.
One study demonstrated that participants underestimated a large meal by up to 1,000 calories. If
you ate an extra 1,000 calories once a week without making up for it with more activity, you
would gain almost 15 pounds in a year. An extra 1,000 calories equate to eating one more slice
of meat lover's pizza and one more fruit smoothie. The bottom line is we eat more than we
think we do, making weight control quite challenging.

WHAT ARE YOU MADE OF?

Muscle Versus Fat
All weight loss is not considered equal. This is a mantra to live by as you embark on your
weight management program. Though we all are conditioned to determine our success solely
by the weight loss shown by the scale, it is much more important to judge our achievements
based on our changes in body composition.

Body Tissues
The human body consists of a variety of diverse types of tissues, lean tissue, and fat tissue. The
lean tissues include bone, muscle, and organs. Muscle and organs are considered metabolically
active, whereas fat is much less metabolically active. This means that muscle and organs help
to increase your metabolism and burn fat and calories, while fat tissue does almost nothing.
Therefore, it is essential to maintain muscle tissue while losing fat, thus the additional
movement will increase your metabolism.

Weight

It is important to realize that a pound of muscle is denser and more compact than a pound of fat. It is helpful to think of a pound of fat as a pound of feathers, and a pound of muscle as a pound of iron. The pound of feathers would clearly take up a lot more space than that same pound of iron. By gaining lean body mass (water, bone, and muscle) while losing body fat, you will look and feel lighter, your clothes will fit better, and your overall sense of well-being will improve. In summary, body weight is only *one* of the many determining factors of success.

Ideal Body Fat Percentage Chart (American Council on Exercise)		
Category	Women	Men
Essential Fat	10-12%	2-4%
Athletes	14-20%	6-13%
Fitness	21-24%	14-17%
Acceptable	25-31%	18-25%
Obese	32+%	26%+

Changing Your Body Composition

To decrease your percent of body fat, you need to create the right balance between the calories you consume and the calories you expend. The most effective way to do this is to decrease your consumption of calories and increase your activity level.

Do what the experts say

The more detailed, consistent, and reliable your information is the easier it is to do your calorie detective work if/when a setback arises. To avoid calorie amnesia, jot down everything you consume right away. Start to pay attention to the calorie content of the items you choose by reading food labels and looking up the calorie content of restaurant foods and beverages.

Keep in mind that many beverages contain calories so be sure to count your calorie containing liquids (Teas, Coffees, sports drinks, and alcohol). They add up quickly. Use the Internet to learn the calorie content of your favorite and most frequently eaten foods. Humans are creatures of habit, you will get familiar with the items you eat regularly, and measuring will no longer be necessary. The idea is to get educated on how much you eat and to know your "go to" foods.

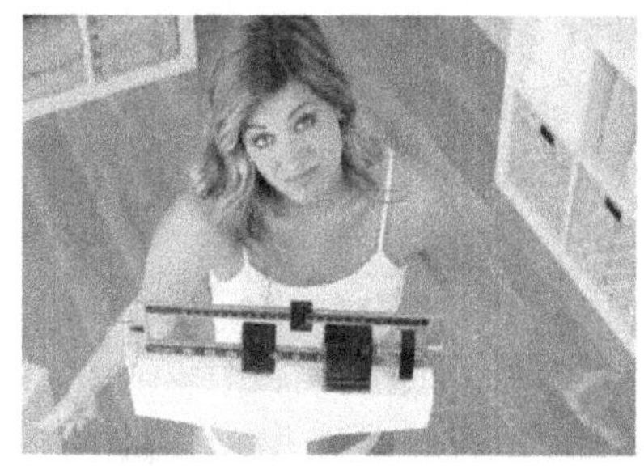

Food **QUANTITY +**
Total **ACTIVITY =**
SCALE WEIGHT

+

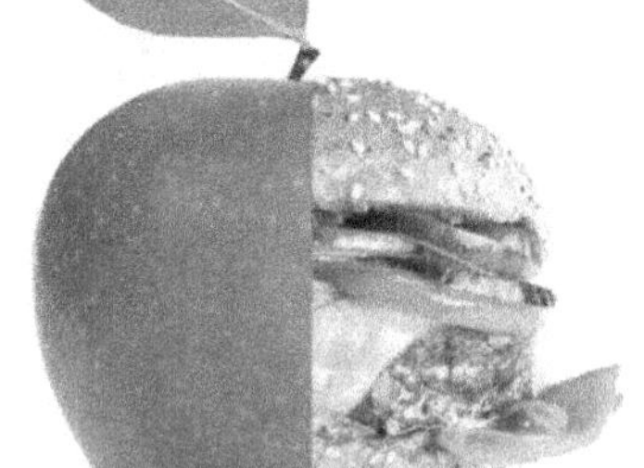

Food **QUALITY +**
WORKOUTS =
Leanness / **BODYFAT %**

+

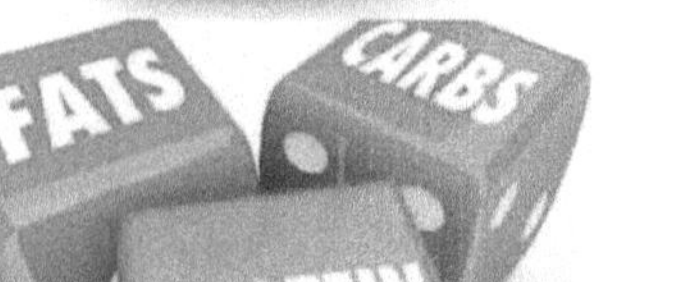

Food **COMBINATIONS =**
Daily **ENERGY, SATIETY**
& PERFORMANCE

= YOUR BODY

Food Logging – A Powerful Weight Loss Tool

Only a small percentage of those who lose at least 10 percent of their initial body weight manage to sustain their results. The remaining majority regain all the weight lost within three to five years. This is likely due to the way many individuals go about losing weight – short-term, or fad diets. The issue with diets is that they tend to be a temporary fix and the eating rules are difficult to sustain. Although you lose weight initially, once you resume your old habits, the weight comes back and there is often more. It is simply unnatural to cut out whole food groups and drastically cut calories - our bodies will fight it. For you to lose weight and keep it off for good, you will have to adjust your food choices and activity level permanently. That means the changes you make should be something you can see yourself doing for the rest of your life. And they do not have to be earth shattering. Perhaps you switch regular soda for diet and save 200 calories a day. And maybe you add a 15-minute walk twice a day and burn 200 more calories, but the bottom line is they are doable for life. Remember, the only proven method to lose weight is to burn more calories than you take in, and research shows that different eating patterns, whether high-carb, low-carb, low-fat or high-fat, can all yield results if you burn more than you take in. Only you can determine what works best for you.

Tips on Food Journaling:

1. **Write as you go.**
   As soon as you eat it, ink it.
2. **Pre-Journal.**
   Write your planned meals/snacks out the night prior. Use a different color pen to check off or write the differences.
3. **Bookend the weekend.**
   Journal on Friday's and Monday's.
   This will keep you on track if you have been doing it a while.

So how do you change or adjust your eating and activity habits? You must first be fully aware of your body's needs and what you are doing now – and you probably aren't. Studies show that most people:

- Do not know how much to eat to maintain their current weight
- Believe they eat less than they do
- Have no idea they take in extra calories in different situations
- Slowly gain 1-3 pounds a year during adulthood until they are overweight or obese

Look for a few things in your journal–

Do I feel more full with meals that have more protein?
Do I feel more full with healthy fats?
Do I feel more full when I get lots of vegetables?
Do I feel more full after quality carbohydrates?
Do I feel extra hungry when I don't get protein?
Do I feel extra hungry when I don't get healthy fats?
Do I feel extra hungry after refined carbohydrates?
Do I feel extra hungry after eating sugar?
Do I feel extra hungry after having juice or soda?
Do I feel extra hungry after missing a meal or an afternoon snack?

Ask those questions of your journal, and let your notes be your guide.

We should always consider things like:

- Am I hungry?
- What am I feeling?
- What are my values?
- What's the situation?
- How unique is this situation?

The solution to becoming aware of your food choices and how much you are eating is to simply pay attention by tracking everything you consume. When you track what you eat, you can't help but notice the types of foods you're eating, the calories in those items, and how your choices affect your weight, appetite and energy levels. By tracking your calories and foods, it becomes clear when you need to make an adjustment. Without knowing what and how much you are eating – it is difficult to make educated decisions. For example, if your daily calorie budget is 1,600 and you eat 1,000 for breakfast, you know you have 600 left for the rest of the day. At this point it is clear that you're probably eating too many calories at breakfast and it's wise to adjust your food choices. You can adjust the portion size of that meal or the choose different foods that have fewer calories and hopefully more nutrients. Again, it is your decision.

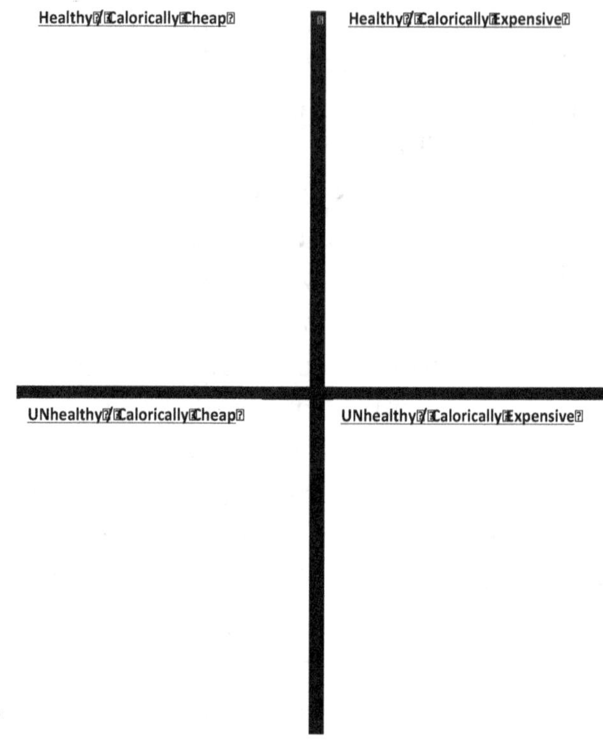

If you still need a reason to track your calories, here it is – you will get twice the results. A large study spanning almost 3 years showed that people who kept tabs of their daily food intake lost twice as much weight as those who did not. Currently, where food is everywhere any time of day and in very large quantities, you can't afford to be unconscious of your choices. By paying attention to portion sizes, calories, and nutrients in foods, you become equipped with new knowledge and therefore, new power to reach and maintain your goals. It is true that knowledge is power, but only if you use that knowledge by taking action.

Time of Day	What I Ate	Hunger Level	Physical Feeling	Emotional Feeling	Thought I Was Thinking	Reason that Thought May Not Be True

Your Plan: For Now, or Forever?

Your habits determine your outcomes. Determining what you can do forever, not just for now, is important. Can you eliminate or drastically reduce foods that you like from your diet? Will you not drink any alcohol ever again? Can you exercise daily for hours for the rest of your life? Will you always rely on prepackaged foods in cardboard boxes?

We have had experience with thousands of individuals, many of which that had or wanted to attempt these "cures" for their unwanted weight gain. Some of these people got very lucky and succeeded with their chosen method but most (98%) are not successful at keeping their weight off for more than one month or two…

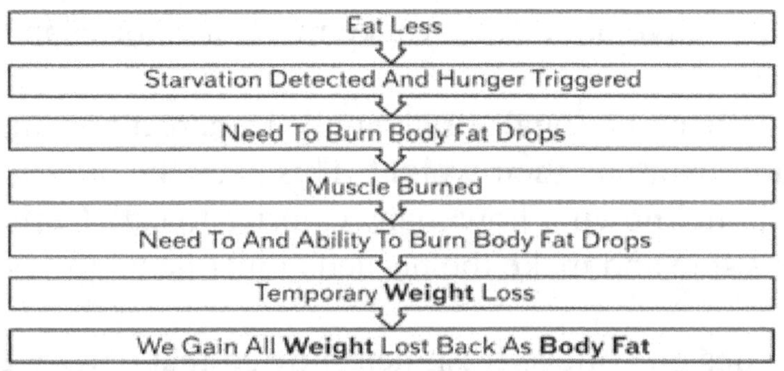

Do you recall back in the 1990's we were told to eat all of the carbohydrates we wanted to as long as we avoided Fat at all costs? We have been told that we can lose all of our weight very quickly if we just don't eat after 8:00PM, we have been told to make sure we combine our meals a certain way and to never eat other foods together. We have been told to eliminate entire food groups, eat like our Paleolithic ancestors did, eat only specific foods, enjoy limitless miracle foods and to exercise as soon as we wake up in the morning or just by exercising our stomachs for 7 minutes a day, we will miraculously look how we want… I believe the reason we fall prey to these "cures" is timing. We are disgusted with ourselves and very, very motivated to change our appearance.

An obstacle we have faced up until now has been that we (as a society) have had little to no solid understanding of all the reasons for weight gain or the best strategies for weight loss. We have had to rely on half-truths and false promises. For many years, I have watched people struggle with understanding why they just cannot diet, eat less for a while and then go back to the way they were living before and expect the results to remain.

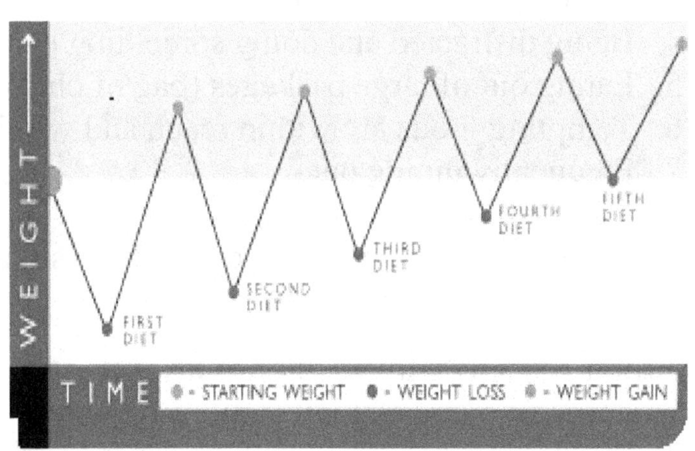

At this point in time we have successfully "blamed" every imaginable thing for our consistent weight gain. We continue to search for the "magic bullet" reason as to why we have gained weight. We have at one point or another blamed every macronutrient, we have blamed our genetics, we have blamed our lifestyle and our lack of control, we have blamed our lack of time and we have blamed our spouses. The consistency is we search externally and continue to assess blame to one thing. It is easier for us to digest (pun ☺) and simpler to comprehend.

However, the reason we gain weight is not simply *one* thing, it is a *cumulative* result of all our habits and behaviors over a lifetime.

What you do not know WILL hurt you
Research shows that most people:
1. Do not know how much to eat to control their weight
2. Do not accurately judge the calories they take in and
3. Have no idea they take in extra calories in different situations.

In a recent national survey, only 15 percent accurately estimated how many calories they should eat to maintain their weight. This begs the question – is it possible to maintain a healthy weight without knowing how many calories to eat? Certainly, if you keep regular tabs on your waistline and make the needed adjustments to your diet or activity level.

Studies on college freshmen showed that daily weighing helped maintain body weight whereas those who did not weigh daily gained nearly seven pounds in ten weeks. Since most people do not weigh themselves daily or even monthly, they do not notice the weight creeping on. And as you can see, what you do not know WILL hurt you. Innovation Fitness suggests self-weighing once per week to avoid weight gain creeping up on you.

When you eat more and do not even realize it
Studies have also shown that we tend to eat more calories in the following situations:
1. Food is presented in copious quantities (restaurants, parties)
2. A wide variety of food is present (buffets, all you can eat)
3. More people are present
4. Being distracted and doing something else (watching TV)
5. Eating out of large packages (bag of chips, tub of ice cream)
6. Tempting foods are within reach and within eyesight
7. Frequently dining out

By becoming aware of how you eat in these situations, you will be better equipped to control the amount of food you take in.

Common reasons why we do not lose weight:
1. Many of our social interactions include food
2. Restaurants portions have increased (particularly fast food)
3. We are less active than in the past
4. We find it unacceptable to be hungry
5. We misunderstand how bodyweight is maintained
6. We forget the extra food we eat every day, or think we ate less than we did
7. We make "poor", reactive decisions surrounding food
8. We fail to plan meals and find ourselves unprepared very often

Practical solutions to start living a healthy, fat loss lifestyle –

1. Stop constantly trying to eat less. Instead eat more fruits, vegetables, and protein more often.
2. Stop exercising more. Begin exercising more efficiently by doing more weight training, less cardio and more leisure walking, which lowers cortisol (your stress hormone) and does not increase appetite.
3. Sleep more by turning off the TV and getting to bed earlier. Health, fitness, and fat loss is more important than your favorite show.... or is it?
4. Stop counting calories and instead measure your control of hunger, energy and cravings and eat to control them so you don't eat more of the wrong things later because you did not eat enough of the correct things earlier.
5. Repeat these steps until it becomes habit.

<u>Remember this equation:</u>

- + - = -   **A negative plus a negative has only one outcome.**
- + + = ?   **A negative plus a positive has multiple outcomes.**
+ + + = +   **Ideal. Be positive and surround yourself with positive support.**

Get informed and take charge

One of the most effective ways to get informed about the way you eat is to track it regularly. To avoid calorie amnesia, jot down everything you consume right away. Start to pay attention to the calorie content of the items you choose by reading food labels and looking up the calorie content of restaurant foods and beverages. Keep in mind that many beverages contain calories so be sure to count those tea drinks, sports drinks, and alcohol. They add up quickly, especially if you are thirsty. In certain states, it is now required by law to post the calorie content directly on the menu board.

What are the top three areas where people go wrong with their eating?

1. Over-Thinking and Creating Complex "Rules"
   Keep it simply, flexible, and real.

2. Under-Feeling and Tuning Out Body Cues
   Sense in, physically, to your body and your biological needs.

3. Giving Eating Too Much Gravity and Shrinking Their Perspective
   Don't lose the big picture. When you over-focus on food, eating habits, and body image, you don't get what you really want, which is to feel good in your body, soul, and spirit.

You will think twice once you realize your favorite coffee drink and muffin has 1,000 calories. If you are really motivated, weigh and measure the amount of food you eat with a food scale, measuring cups and measuring spoons and calculate the calories you take in. Since humans are creatures of habit, you will get familiar with the items you eat regularly, and measuring will no longer be necessary. The idea is to get educated on how much you eat.

> **Be Solution Based, not Problem Based.**
> **It is easy to give up. It takes strength, commitment, and dedication to persevere.**
> **Begin to think about your possibilities – not your limitations.**

To prevent unconsciously eating excess calories, follow these tips:
- Eat and only eat- avoid being distracted during mealtimes or snack times
- Eat from smaller plates, bowls, and glasses
- Portion out your food and avoid "family style" eating or eating out of the package
- When you dine out, control the portion sizes by sharing meals or packaging some to take home right away
- During social occasions, decide on what you are going to eat and stick to it- otherwise you will graze mindlessly
- Limit your alcohol intake- alcohol tends to stimulate appetite and reduce your awareness of what you are eating and how much
- Keep snacks, treats and tempting foods out of reach
- The adage "knowledge is power" is true for weight control if you use it to make informed decisions

It is not rocket science if you judge RESULTS over time
It is challenging to manage something you are not aware of and do not keep track of. Since only one third of the population acknowledges that calories are responsible for weight gain, it is no wonder there is an obesity epidemic. And by the way, it is no coincidence that one third of adults have a healthy body weight. Knowing how much you consume is a key part of successful weight control, but even if you do not know – the scale will tell you. If the number on your scale increases over time, (month to month – NOT day to day) you are taking in more calories than you are burning – PERIOD. The solution is to burn off that extra fuel by moving more and eating fewer calories. If you do not measure your results by checking your weight regularly, you will end up sabotaging your waistline and likely your health too.

The compound effect on weight loss
One of the most dangerous traps that you can fall into while dieting is having the "All or Nothing" attitude. Therefore, many people who are trying to lose weight fail at their attempts. They make a mistake here and there, whether that is missing a day of exercise or indulging in treats too frequently and end up so discouraged that they just give up completely. Losing sight of the big picture is deadly if you are on a weight loss journey. But it is sometimes hard to see the big picture when you get mired down in the day-to-day grind of little decisions. The truth is that everybody fails sometimes. Everybody. If you expect perfection from yourself, you will certainly be disappointed, because it is not possible.

You see, focusing on occasional failures is like looking at snapshots rather than the entire movie. If you went to see a movie that was two hours in length, you would see a whole story complete with plot, background, character development, suspense, and conclusion. In other words, you would come away with a full scope of the big picture.

But suppose your friend, rather than seeing the movie, only saw a handful of still shots from it. Would your perception be different? Of course, it would. You might even disagree about what happened in the movie. This is because she can only focus on a few aspects of the movie, whereas you can see the big picture. Sure, the main character might have made a mistake at some point, or perhaps things looked bad for part of the movie, but that is only part of the movie. It is not the final outcome.

Looking at your own journey to health in the same way is critical if you are going to get through the bad days and the periods of discouragement. Your failures are only a still shot within a fully developed screenplay. The extra dessert you ate yesterday is a snapshot, it is not the whole picture. The whole picture includes the one hundred times last month that you **resisted** unhealthy food!

Therefore, the compound effect is so helpful when you are making hard lifestyle changes. Every single good decision you make adds up to a magnificent outcome. Sure, maybe you did skip your workout three times last week. Okay, that happens; it was a rough week. But remember how many workouts you have accomplished over the last six months? Remember how you took the stairs instead of the elevator several times last week?

Healthy choices compound to create a tapestry of health improvement and weight control. They are cumulative. They are the movie, not the snapshot. You will fall occasionally. Just pick yourself up, acknowledge that you are not perfect, remind yourself of how far you have come and file that snapshot away. **<u>You do not need it</u>**: you have an entire movie to watch.

Your changes and habits must fit your goal
Often, I hear from new client, and multiple people daily, that they "Eat Healthy" and I do not doubt it. Many health and weight conscious people tend to eat healthier than those that are not. Also, people in transition (dieting etc.…) tend to make better, healthier food choices.

However, I often find that people have a clear misunderstanding of what it means to eat and train for a specific goal. Common thinking is that one style of eating or training will translate into the desired goal. Let us be clear – this is NOT the truth. Specific actions determine specific outcomes and just because you want something to happen does not mean that it will.

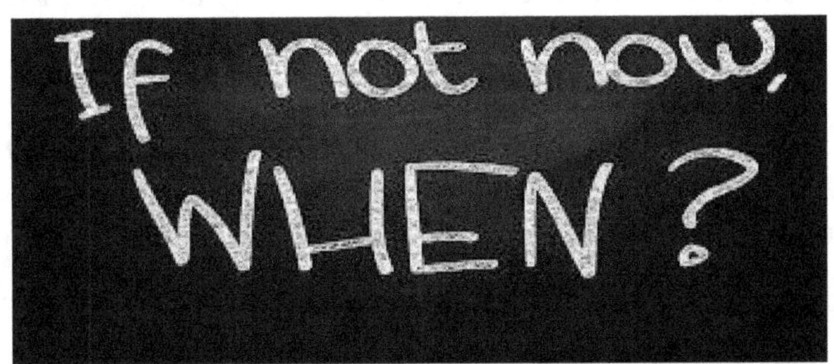

Understanding Scale Weight Fluctuations

WHY does this happen?
There are two things you need to be familiar with. The first is essential body mass (EBM). Your body is made up of a bunch of things like bones, muscles, organs, tissues, skin, etc. These are essential, and you *cannot* lose them. It is not like you will cut off your femur to drop a few pounds. They are on or in your body and cannot be taken out to affect the scale weight.

The second thing you need to understand is your Lean Body Mass (LBM). Your lean body mass is the amount of weight you carry on your body that is not fat. The goal is to drop weight while keeping your lean body mass the same, or in other words, dropping your body fat percentage. This is also the driving factor of your metabolism. For it to function efficiently, you need a greater amount of LBM. To understand these fluctuations, we are going to focus on the 3 things that add to your body weight. They are fat, muscle, and water.

Fat
Your body *needs* fat. However, if you have an energy imbalance (more energy coming in rather than going out) you can store more fat than needed. The goal is to be in a healthy negative energy balance so that you lose weight.

Muscle
Your body has muscle (if it did not you would not be able to move) and obviously the more you work out the more muscle you can gain, thus increasing your weight. Muscle is denser than fat, so it takes up less space. It is true, 10 lbs. of muscle = 10 lbs. of fat HOWEVER it is much more compact/dense than fat.

Water
Your body needs water. It is made up of 60% water, which is crucial for your body to function properly. It transports nutrients, oxygen, and waste in and out of cells. Drink it. Fat, muscle, and water are the three things that cause weight changes on the scale.

Here is a simple hypothetical
Let us say someone is 140lbs of lean body mass (LBM) and 40 lbs. of fat. They would weigh 180 lbs. and have a body fat percentage of 22.22%. This person steps on the scale one day and it is 180 lbs. The next day it is 182, and the following day it is 179. I know you have seen this with your weight, and you are probably wondering why it happens. Here is a formula that can explain that.

> ***Scale weight = True Weight +/- weight variance (the daily change that occurs)***

True Weight = Hypothetical perfect weight if there was such a thing. It is essentially exactly what you would weigh minus all the issues that cause weight variations.

Weight Variance= All the daily changes.

4 Factors That Cause Weight Scale Fluctuations

1. Glycogen

Your body breaks down the carbohydrates that you eat into a type of sugar called glucose, which is your main source of energy. When your body has too much glucose it stores the leftover in your liver and muscles. The stored form of glucose (in your liver and muscles) is called glycogen.

Each gram of glycogen is bound by about four grams of water. This means when your liver and muscles are full of glycogen you can gain four times the weight of that glycogen in water.

More glycogen = More water

When you diet and cut carbs, your body empties out those stored carbohydrates from the liver and muscles. When you lose that glycogen, you lose that water. That is why when you start a low carb diet you lose weight quickly (anywhere from 2-10 pounds based on your size). When you start to eat carbs again, your liver and muscles will take that glucose and replenish the stock. Once it does that, four grams of water joins the glycogen and voila, you gain weight back. So, if you gain 5 pounds on the scale 24-48 hours after binge eating, that would probably be your explanation. You did not suddenly gain 5 pounds of "fat."

2. Food Weight

This one might be common sense, but many forget. Food has a specific weight. 1 pound of chicken weighs 1 pound. 1 pint of water weighs 1 pound. So, if you were to eat a pound of chicken and immediately step on the scale you would gain 1 pound. Food and water will adjust your weight. If you eat a huge Thanksgiving Day meal and immediately step on the scale you will have an increase in weight. To go a bit farther, everything you eat sits in your digestive tract for at least a day and while it sits there it contributes to the scale weight.

3. Sodium (retaining and depletion)

Sodium is another reason why you experience significant fluctuations on the scale. You might go to a baseball game, eat some nachos, pizza, and sunflower seeds. Your sodium intake is drastically increased compared to a normal day.

When you increase your sodium, you increase a hormone in your body called Aldosterone. Aldosterone affects sodium, potassium, total fluid in the body, and blood pressure. It causes the kidneys to hold on to more sodium, which leads to more water staying in the body. Eating less sodium decreases the production of Aldosterone causing your body to hold on to less water. If this is an issue for you, obviously, limit your sodium intake.

4. Hormonal Issues

This goes for both males and females, but without a doubt the females will see this more often. Typically, when it's that time of month there can be a MAJOR fluctuation in water balance. It can be anywhere from 2-10 lbs. based off the individual. Another major issue is stress. Stress can drastically impact fluid retention and of course, it can lead to poor eating habits causing you to consume more sodium, bad fats, and unnecessary carbohydrates. The obvious answer for this is control your stress levels to better manage this aspect.

What Should You Do?
When you are dieting, you are going to see frequent weight swings. The primary reason is because glycogen is a much more volatile substrate than fat. Fat loss occurs slowly while glycogen levels can swing like crazy (sodium, stress, etc. change hourly as well).

Remember that you are an individual
You might have a friend who can eat anything they want, and never gain an ounce of fat. Why is that? You may know someone who says, "Just looking at food makes me gain weight." Why is that? Each person is a separate individual with their own genetic make-up. There are three body types and metabolisms that are determined by genetics, gender and compliance.

Ectomorph: Someone with a fast metabolism, low set point (fat thermostat), can stay very lean and has a difficult time building muscle.
- Ex. A long distance runner.

Mesomorph: Someone with a medium metabolism, medium set point (fat thermostat), can stay lean and build muscle.
- Ex. A sprinter or wide receiver.

Endomorph: Someone with a slow metabolism, high set point (fat thermostat), can build muscle and store high amounts of body fat.
- Ex. An offensive lineman.

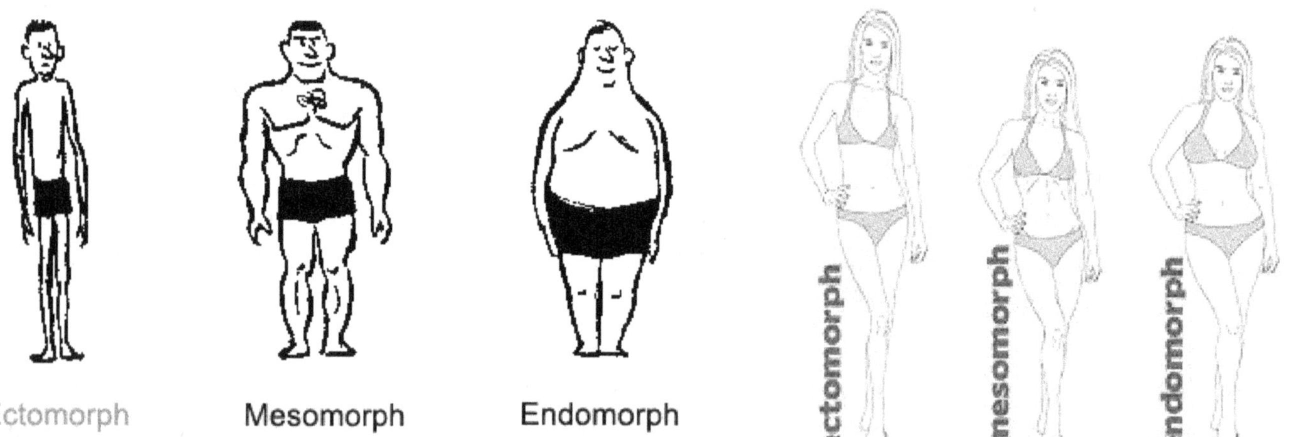

Most of the population has characteristics of each body type. The important thing to understand is that your genetics and gender are determined at birth, and your compliance (the choices you make with your nutrition, fitness and overall health) will help you reprogram your metabolism to achieve your goals. People are gifted in different areas; some have an extremely fast metabolism and never have to think about gaining body fat, some are extremely intelligent, or some have a great sense of humor or deep sense of service. Often, exercise program gimmicks will target your insecurities by suggesting they have unlocked the keys to changing your stubborn areas with their specific set and order of exercises, or their "breakthrough" weight loss plan… Reality tells us a different story. The bottom line is that we all have strengths and challenges. The key to success in nutrition and fitness is to understand YOUR metabolism, and what level of compliance is necessary to teach your body to work for you. Comparing yourself to others will usually lead to disappointment and frustration. Every person can succeed; all you need to do is make the choice.

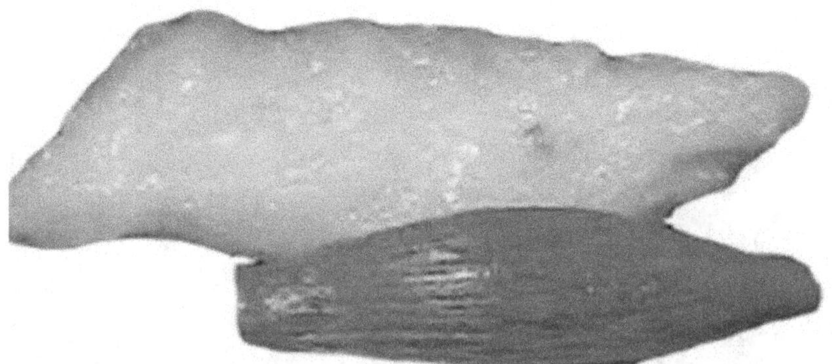

Above are identical replicas of 5 lbs. of fat (yellow) and 5 lbs. of muscle

EATING

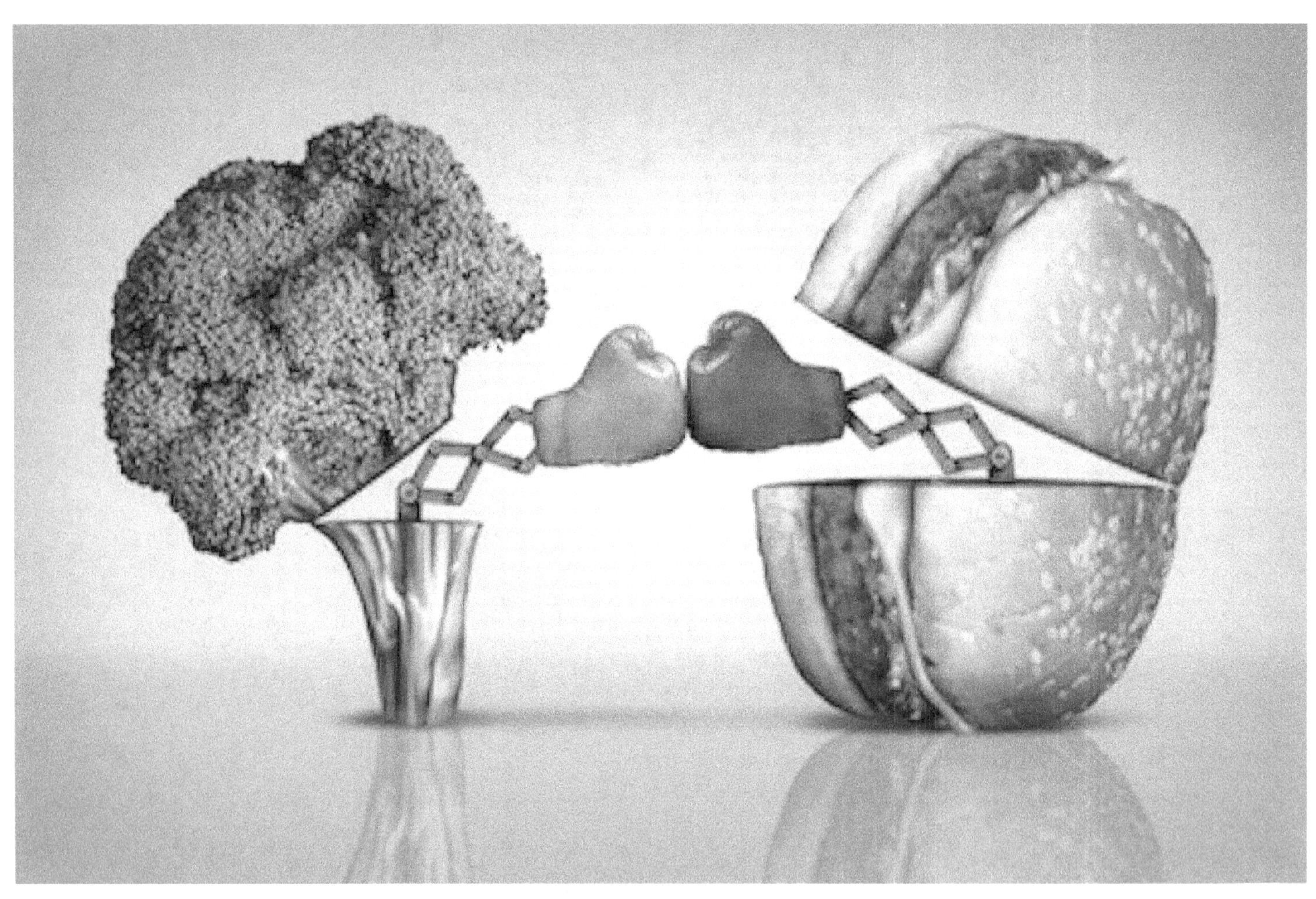

Take stock of your environment and your thought process prior to and during eating times. Create the proper environment and utilize the correct tools for consistent changes.

1. Your Current eating habits.
- Do you eat at desk?
- Where and how do you eat most of your meals?
- What do you eat during these times?
- How will this be compatible with your new food choices?

2. Are you prepared to eat differently than your friends at social functions?
- Eating often accompanies many social gatherings. How do your friends eat?
- Do they consume foods that you know will not be compatible with your lifestyle?
- How will you address this?

3. Are you prepared to change your home environment?
- Does your home environment work with your new plans? You may have chosen to eat mindfully and leisurely. The trouble is your home is utterly chaotic, noisy, and messy, with barely a place to sit down, let alone have a large, pleasant space to indulge in your new meals.
- What will you do to change this?

4. How do your current habits fit?
- What if your leisure activities always involve eating junk food?
- What happens if you start a diet that completely rules out junk food?
- What will you do? Change your habits? Find a different comfort food?

5. What about eating away from home?
- Do you eat at restaurants a lot?
- Which restaurants do you go to?
- Will they fit with your new style of eating?
- Are you prepared to leave food on your plate if their portions are too big?

6. Is your kitchen set-up properly?
- Look around your kitchen.
- Do you have enough fridge/freezer space?
- Do you have proper cookware?
- Do you have enough containers? Enough time?

7. Are you being totally honest with yourself?
- You read about a new diet in a magazine, and it requires eating a lot more vegetables. On the surface you are busting to lose "10 pounds in 2 weeks", but deep down you know you cannot stand vegetables. Which part of you will win out in the end?

- Why do you hate veggies? Are you prepared to cook more, or learn different ways of cooking them?

8. Can you accept the things you cannot change?
- You cannot change the way other people act and the way they speak - "oh, so you're on another health kick, again are you?" But you can choose ahead of time how you will respond inwardly and outwardly.

9. Will you continue monitoring yourself objectively?
- Many people reach their ideal weight, and then let old habits creep back in. However, there are a few warning systems in place. One is the waistband in your pants. Will you choose to conveniently ignore it if it gets tighter? Or will you be objective?

10. How will the lifestyle of family and friends affect your health/weight loss efforts?
- If your entire world is filled with people who are lazy people, how do you plan to work against this culture?
- Will they influence you to be more active or more sedentary?

Planning and measuring for Nutrition Success

Good nutrition achieves health, body composition and performance goals.
Good nutrition is about more than weight loss or gain, since energy balance and weight can change from one day to the next. Therefore, finding a long-term set of dietary habits should be based on the intersection of the following three goals:
1. Improved **body composition**
2. Improved **health**
3. Improved **performance**

Good nutrition properly controls **energy balance, provides nutrient density, and** achieves **health, body composition,** and **performance** goals.

Clear goals, consistent actions and great planning bring about success

Continually ask yourself the following questions:
- What exactly am I trying to achieve?
- What is the exact strategy I am using to achieve it?
- In what areas am I producing the results I desire?
- In what areas am I not producing optimal results?
- Which part of my process is not performing?
- How can I adapt that part of the process so I can test my modified strategy against the desired result?
- What would happen if I completely reinvented my strategy?
- Most important: What can I do right now to help me achieve my goal?

WHAT IS A CALORIE?

CALORIES MEASURE FOOD ENERGY

The amount of calories in our food reflects the amount of
energy that food provides our bodies

THE AMOUNT OF CALORIES IN 1 GRAM OF EACH MACRONUTRIENT

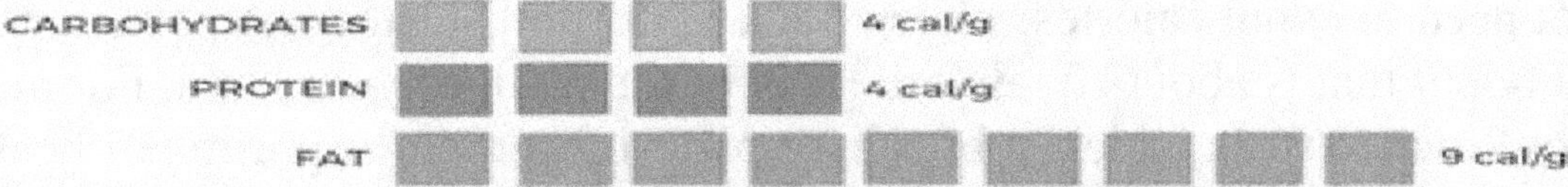

CARBOHYDRATES	PROTEIN	FAT
Main source of fuel and easily used by the body for energy	Essential for growth, tissue repair, immune function, preserving muscle and producing essential hormones	Essential in cell, nerve tissue and hormone production: the most concentrated source of energy

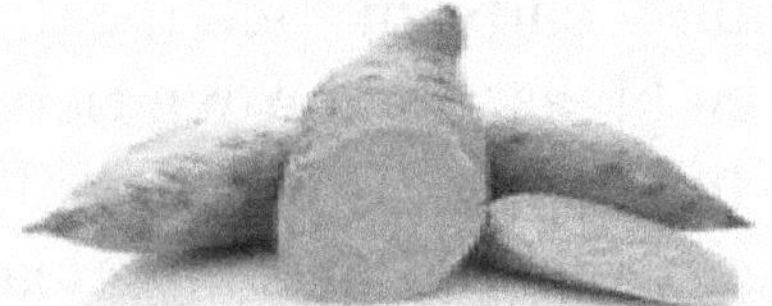

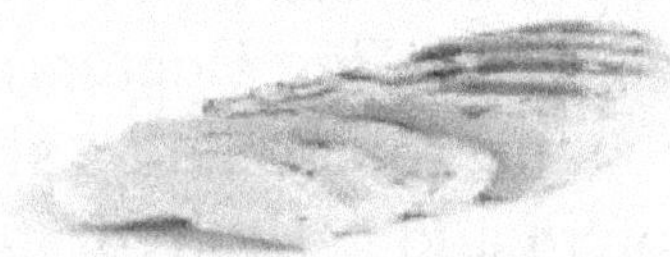

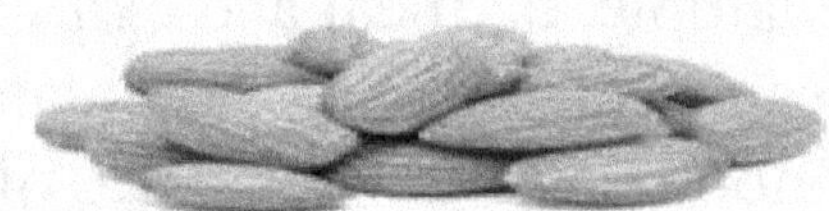

WHAT ARE MACROS?

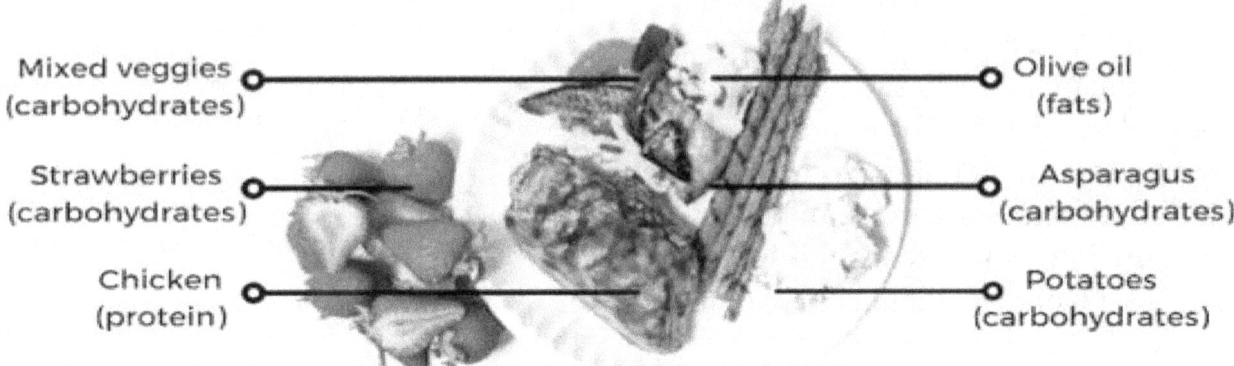

CARBOHYDRATES	PROTEIN	FAT
• 4 calories per gram • provides energy, assists in fat metabolism, prevents protein breakdown • recommended intake 30-40% of daily caloric intake	• 4 calories per gram • provides energy, supports muscle growth & repair • recommended intake: 30-40% of daily caloric intake	• 9 calories per gram • provides energy, absorbs vitamins, regulates body temperature, has essential fatty acids • recommended intake 20-30% of daily caloric intake

The Right FACTS

- **Foods** - The best Foods are high in nutrients and calorie compact. My favorite protein foods are eggs, chicken, salmon, lean beef, low-fat cottage cheese and a Light Nutrition Shake. For carbohydrates, I like baked potato, brown rice, oatmeal, apples, oranges, and strawberries. And for vegetables, I eat a lot of steamed broccoli, spinach, and green beans. You get the idea.
- **Amounts** - The next key is to eat the correct amounts of those healthy foods I mentioned above. I do not need to count calories; I keep track of portions instead. A portion of protein is an amount that is about equal to the size of the palm of your hand. For me, that is about an 8 or 9-ounce steak, chicken breast, or piece of salmon. A portion of healthy carbs is an amount approximately equal to the size of your closed hand. For me, that is a good-sized baked potato, about 1.25 cups of cooked brown rice or cooked oatmeal. For vegetables, the portion rule is how much you can pile into your cupped hand. I can stack it high, so I have large servings of steamed broccoli very often with my dinners.
- **Combinations** - Now we need the Right Combinations of the Right Foods, in the Right Amounts. I combine a portion of protein and a portion of healthy carbs in each meal. For example, oatmeal and egg whites (I like Egg Beaters), chicken breast and brown rice; lean steak and a baked potato; cottage cheese and a sliced, whole apple. It is especially important to get a balance of protein and carbohydrates in every one of our daily meals.
- **Times** - The correct Time to eat. - Feeding the body on a schedule of every 3.5 – 5 hours is ideal. This schedule allows you to stabilize your blood sugar and energy levels, minimize cravings and appetite and helps ensure our bodies have a constant supply of the healthy nutrients needed to support health and fitness. We also have better digestion and more energy when we eat smaller meals frequently throughout the day.

Get your FACT's straight

As you might imagine, the best combination of nutrient and calorie density for improving health and promoting fat loss is a diet **high in nutrient-dense foods** (a lot of nutrients- vitamins, minerals, fiber- per calorie) and **low in calorie-dense foods** (few calories per gram of food weight). Such a diet would have the following benefits:

- Easily controlled calorie intake (without calorie counting)
- Longer periods of **satiation**, or satisfaction/fullness, after meals
- Difficulty overeating
- A higher total essential nutrient intake
- More essential nutrients per volume of food

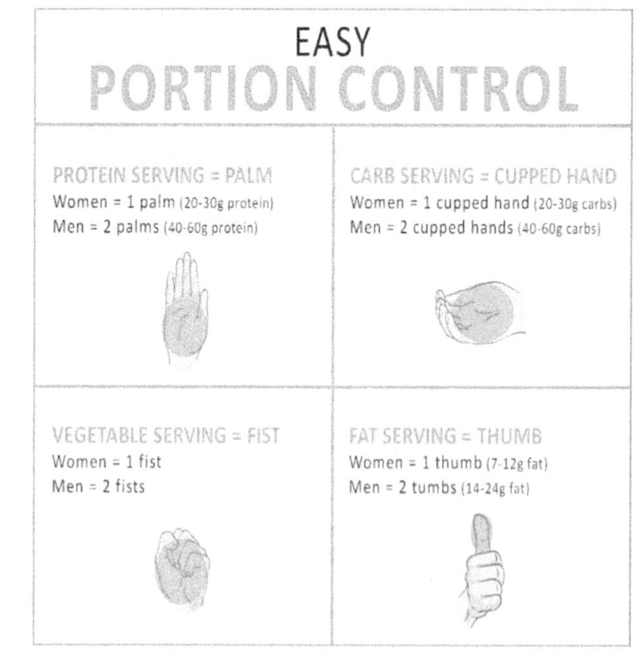

The perfect diet is created, not found, and the journey is what allows the creation process to unfold. The four guideposts are:

1. Is your CHEC in check?
CHEC stands for Control of Cravings, Hunger and Energy. These four parameters are feedback clues for you to conduct your detective work with. Balancing, or learning to control these factors is critical if you are going to turn any diet into a lifestyle. Assess CHEC weekly, assigning a scale of 1-10 to hunger, cravings, and energy. 10 being high and 1 being low.
- Hunger and cravings should be less than 5
- Energy should be 6 or more

2. Are you losing fat?
Remember, weight loss and fat losses are **not** the same. You could be losing weight and be losing a considerable amount of water, or worse - muscle, rather than fat. After CHEC is stable, make sure you are measuring fat loss. If you are losing mostly fat, then you are doing great.

3. Is your health improving?
There are 3 main reasons people go on a diet and exercise program in the first place…
1. To look good.
2. To feel good.
3. To live longer.

With CHEC balanced you will likely feel better than you have in a long-time. If you are losing fat you are going to look better too. You also want to know if you are making a difference in health and longevity. For that, it is about your health numbers (resting heart rate, cholesterol levels, lipid profiles etc.…) and clinical signs and symptoms. Is your blood pressure improving? Is your heart rate decreasing? Is your blood sugar more balanced? Are you sleeping better without snoring? Is your doctor happy with your blood lab numbers?

4. Is your performance improving?
If your diet is creating a calorie deficit, but your energy is dwindling and your workout effort and/or desire to workout suffers, do you believe that it is serving its' purpose? Your diet should energize your workout efforts and recovery. It should improve your workout performance, serve to increase strength levels and your ability to complete tasks of daily living.

If all these above factors are true, you have created the perfect lifestyle for you. If they are not, you will need to evaluate which aspects of your dietary intake are serving these outcomes and which need to be revised. Your ultimate diet is a lifestyle in which you see these four components improve and allows for satiety and satisfaction from your food intake.

5 Questions for Fat Loss

Most people have heard about how to eat for fat loss, but they just cannot figure out what to eat when it comes time for a meal. That is largely because they are asking themselves the wrong questions. It helps if you ask the right questions at the most critical time – when it is time to pick up the fork and spoon.

1. Are you eating too much food?

When fat loss is your primary goal, you should stop eating when you are about **80% full**. This will leave you satiated but not belly-rubbing full. So, for this next meal, do you plan on eating a little less than you normally would? You can eat from a smaller plate than usual. You can leave a little on the plate, instead of finishing everything in front of you. Or you can stop at one serving instead of going back for seconds. Whatever strategy you use, make sure you are decreasing your calories compared to what you might normally eat.

2. Are you eating enough protein?

Your protein intake determines whether you are going to lose body fat or lean muscle, obviously, we want to lose the first and keep the latter. So, for this next meal, is there enough lean protein included? Men should eat about 2 palm-sized portions and women should eat about 1 palm-sized portion. You can choose from sources including lean meats (chicken, turkey, fish, lean beef, lean game meats), lean vegetarian sources (tofu, tempeh, legumes), or powdered protein supplements. Whichever you choose, make sure you are eating more protein than what you might normally eat.

3. Are you eating too many sugars or starches?

Too many starches and sugars in your diet can prevent fat loss (or even cause fat gain). So, for this next meal, are there too many starches, particularly processed ones like bread or pasta? Men should eat less than 1 fist-sized portion and women should eat less than ½ fist-sized portion. Also, the amount of sugar should be minimized.

Starches in the diet include grains, pasta, potatoes, rice, bread, and other carb-dense foods. And added sugars can be found in pop/soda, fruit juices, salad dressings, desserts, sweet snacks, and more. Again, you do not have to cut these out completely. You just must be sure to eat fewer of them than usual.

4. Are you eating enough vegetables?

By replacing your grains with greens, you will still feel satisfied at the end of a meal while also increasing your intake of fiber and other important vitamins/minerals. So, for this next meal, are you eating enough vegetables? For fat loss, men should eat about 1 cup while women should eat about ½ cup. While most people think of salads when veggies are brought up, many other options are available. Baked, grilled, sautéed, or steamed veggies all count. As do foods like pesto or even kale chips. Regardless of which veggies you choose, make sure you are eating more than usual.

5. Are you including enough healthy fats?
Highly processed fats, trans and saturated, often found in processed foods, can ruin your health and lead to fat gain. However, a healthy mix of other naturally occurring fats is important for fat loss. So, for this next meal, are you eating some healthy unsaturated fats?

You can choose from sources like olive oil, avocados, raw nuts (not roasted), raw seeds, and omega-3 rich fish oils. Whichever you choose, make sure you are adding healthy fats to your diet while replacing the unhealthy ones.

Here are some food suggestions that will fill you up without filling you out:
- Large salad with romaine lettuce, tomatoes, cucumber, carrots, red cabbage, broccoli, shredded cheese, sunflower seeds, whole grain croutons, and pecans. Dressing: lightly sprinkle with olive oil and balsamic vinegar
- Quinoa salad: chilled quinoa, sliced avocado, diced tomato, onion, lemon juice and salt
- Whole grain rye cracker with nut butter spread
- Baked sweet potato with chopped pecans
- Wild rice seasoned with dried garlic, onion and freshly ground black pepper
- Slow cooked beans (pinto, black, navy, etc.) with a sprinkling of grated cheese
- High fiber fruit: apples, pears, grapefruit, figs
- Whole grain breads
- Protein shakes with frozen berries and frozen kale
- Cut up vegetables dipped in Greek Yogurt

Anytime you begin to feel hungry, choose from the above list to ease your hunger and gain a feeling of satiety. Your diet stress will ease, and you will be more likely to stick to it in the long term!

What are the three biggest obstacles I'm going to run into with food?

1. ____
2. ____
3. ____

What are three structures I can put in place to overcome those three obstacles?

1. ____
2. ____
3. ____

What should you eat?

Food Rules for Fat Loss

1. For weight loss, your most important task is to eat things that help you create a calorie deficit.

- **For sports nutrition**: your most important task is to eat foods that help you take in enough energy, carbohydrates, and protein for optimal performance and recovery.
- **For disease prevention**: you want to choose foods that are high in some nutrients, and low in others
- **For mending a disordered relationship with food:** follow the guidelines for everyone, eat some of everything, and do not let your brain get wrapped up in details of what foods you choose. Stay focused on how much and why you are eating Schedule your Fat Loss

2. Plan and *schedule your fat loss training* in line with your physical training. This is intelligent and sustainable. You cannot be on a fat loss plan all the time. Fat loss slows down and eventually stops, making your efforts futile and counterproductive.

- Follow the Fat Loss Guidelines during STRENGTH – BURN
- Follow Metabolism Boosting Guidelines during STRENGTH – BUILD

3. Exit Strategy

Always have an *exit strategy* for the plan you are currently doing. If you are attempting a plan for X numbers of days, what is your plan after day X? Know what you will do after, do not wait until day X + 1 to figure it out. Typically, people choose diets due to being in an unhappy state. They commit to "all or none" protocols and when willpower gives out, which it ALWAYS does, they are left with no plan, causing major rebounds in weight and mental fatigue.

By aligning and periodizing your training and nutrition, you gain a timeline and an exit strategy for your current plan. Remember that nothing works forever; so, attempting to constantly lose fat is a lose/lose situation. As a matter of fact, studies show that chronic dieting causes long-term fat/weight gain.

During STRENGTH – BUILD periods, you should increase your calorie intake to increase strength and muscle tissue. Remember, muscle is what allows you to increase your metabolism, look toned, and eat more food. Muscle is what makes people look athletic. Muscle is the **primary driver of your metabolism**.

- During STRENGTH - **BUILD** months: when you increase food do not add junk calories. Maintain food quality; just eat slightly more (200-300 calories).
- During STRENGTH – **BURN** months: you would reduce Total Calorie Intake (TCI) by 200-300 calories per day. Food Quality will remain high.

4. Nutrition first, calories second

The greatest gift you can give your body is to improve the quality of your food. Better quality of food will result in a leaner, stronger body, regardless of your goal. The goal is to eat as many high nutrition, high volume, and low-calorie foods as possible.

IFS Nutrition Targets allow you to control your calorie intake without having to count them. It allows for nutrition to be the priority and for calorie control to occur as a byproduct of eating better.

Target	Minimum	Ideal
Protein	.5 oz/lb of body weight	.75 oz/lb of body weight
Water	.5 oz/lb of body weight	.75 oz/lb of body weight
Fiber		35+ grams/day Veggies and berries first. Whole grains last.

5. Simple AND Effective

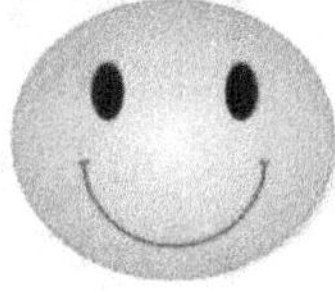

- Calorie counting is accomplished by achieving and maintaining these targets. Remember there are PLENTY of things to eat, but not a lot of food choices in our current environment.
- Green-face rule- if it has a face or is green (or purple, red, or orange) then eat it. Simple.
- Avoid cardboard carbs- if it is bleached, processed, comes out of a cardboard box or is "food-like," but not actual food, then do not bother eating it.
- Invest in a quality protein supplement, meal replacement formula, and greens blend (dotfit lean MR, Vega one essentials)
    - Recipe - Begin with a MRF base, add the greens blend to the shake mix container and if you do not eat many healthy fats, you should add flax/chia seeds to the blend. Do it once to simplify your life.

	CARBS	PROTEIN	FAT
Aim To Eat	• Whole grain bread • Oats • Pumpkin • Mixed vegetables • Squash • Whole wheat crackers • Low-fat popcorn • Beans and Lentils • All fruits • Low-fat milk and yogurt • Brown rice	• Eggs • Cottage cheese • Skinless chicken and turkey • Reduced- fat cheese • Nuts and nut butters • Non-fried fish • Rice and beans	• Avocado • Nuts and nut butters • Canola oil • Olive oil • Pumpkin seeds • Sunflower seeds
Okay in Moderation	• Regular granola • Bagels • Dinner rolls • Cold cereals	• Light sausage • Low-fat beef and pork	• Regular salad dressing • Mayonnaise • Butter or margarine • Canned olives
Limit Intake	• Soda • Fruit juices • Cake • Brownies • Cookies, pie, candy • Gravy, stuffing	• Bacon • Regular fat cheese • Hot dogs • Processed sandwich meat • High-fat sausage and beef • Protein powders	• Shortening or anything with hydrogenated oils • Bacon • Sour cream

6. Control your environment

- **If you do not have it, you cannot eat it**- this goes for nutritious and non-nutritious food.
  - Be sure to grocery shop. Have prepared foods and meals ready to go.
- **Speed** – the speed of eating is a prime determining factor in how many calories you eat in any feeding. People who slow down, savor their food, and do not speed eat tend to eat up to 25% less calories per meal. Bonus- this will aid in digestion.
- **Eat breakfast**- people who eat breakfast, specifically with added protein, tend to have fewer energy crashes and eat up to 30% less in total daily calories.
- **Eat by the clock, not by your stomach** - know what, when, and where your next meal is. Never wait until you are hungry. Like Snickers says, you are not you when you are hungry. You will eat whatever does not outrun you.
- **Plan, shop, prepare, cook, eat**- when you meal plan, begin with your proteins and veggies. Then add your carbohydrates based on your activity needs and goals. Be sure to shop for good, quality food and take time to plan what, where, and when you will eat.
- **Eating order**- eat your vegetables first, protein second, and save your starchy carbohydrates for last. During BURN months, at least twice per week, attempt to have double-veggies and no starches for dinner. Be sure not to go starch free on workout days and to schedule your non-starch days for non-workout days only. No "double-carbing." If your big picture goals include attaining and maintaining a lean and healthy physique, there are very few times that you "need" to double-carb.
  1. Example 1- there is no need to have pasta and bread in the same meal.
  2. Example 2- a burrito is a triple carb (the wrap, rice, and beans)
  3. Example 3- mashed potatoes and corn (corn and potatoes are considered grains, not vegetables)

Simple Meal Creator

PROTEIN	VEGGIES	STARCH	FAT	FLAVOR
MEALS				

7. Track it

If you think it, you ink it. If you don't, you won't. A food journal is an extremely reliable accountability tool. Accuracy aside, the accountability of having to be raw and honest with each feeding and having the ability for a Professional to review to find Nutritional and Habit gaps is essential.

- No need to overwhelm yourself. Commit to 2 weekdays and 1 weekend day per month for 1 month. Repeat this every other month.

8. 3S model

Meals should supply nutrition, but also be palatable and match your eating style. Ideally, they should be enjoyable. Fullness leads to Fat Loss.

- Satiety- Should fill you
- Satisfaction- Satisfy your taste buds
- Sustainability- You can keep doing it

9. Measure

Cost vs Value- spend 10-15 minutes extra on a task to save 15 minutes x 10 extra there.

- Cook large, package small. When you cook, be sure to make as many meals at once as possible.
- Cook 10 meals
  - Eat now
  - Put in the fridge
  - Put in the freezer (labeled)
- Tip: for more freshness, cook 2x a week instead of just one. Maybe Monday and Wednesday work better for your schedule and preferences.
- Tip: make crock-pot bags of raw ingredients, wake up, toss in the bag and move on with your day, knowing that Dinner will be ready.
- If you do not like preparing food, there are services that can help you with that:
  - Buying precut vegetables at the grocery store
  - Buy precut meats at the grocery store
  - Take advantage of services that deliver all ingredients ready to cook
  - Taking the extra time to cook in advance will save hours later and help to make better food decisions
- Meal prepping will help reduce stress and save time

10. STOP THE JUSTIFICATIONS

- Ask yourself why you are eating something (out loud) before eating.
- "Because I want it" "Because I earned it" etc.
- Challenge "I want", instead ask "based on my actions, what do I need?"

11. Make better bad choices
Increase Surprise Exercise and
Minimize Damage

- **First rule of weight loss**: drink more water and sleep more. Two non-caloric actions that will decrease cravings, boost energy and speed metabolism.
- Get up and move throughout the day.
- Make your next best choice. Leave your poor choices in the past.

Food Habits

1. **Always have water available** - take a drink while you think. It will help to prevent poor decisions and decrease calorie intake.
2. **Have convenient foods available**- frozen meals (IFS approved = Kashi, EVOL, Nurture Bowls, Power Bowls), healthy food bars, microwavable foods, and Steamed Veggies (for when you are in a hurry or have not planned and are hungry). For a more filling and healthier frozen meal, add veggies to it.
3. **Plate your food**- if you stand while you eat or eat while you prep, then eat again you can expect your calories to skyrocket.
4. **Minimize Liquid calories**- hot beverages, teas, sports drinks, juices etc.…
5. **"Don't let perfect get in the way of better"**- You will not achieve perfection and you will make poor food choices. One bad meal or bad day does not "blow it".
6. **Focus on what you can do, not on what you cannot**- Health, Wellness and Weight Loss is a lifelong process. Take it one step at a time.
7. **Know that you are doing good things for yourself** - Focus on what you are gaining, not on what you are losing. What does eating "better" add to your life?
8. **Caloric restriction without calorie quality is a recipe for disaster.**

Mindful Eating Journal

TRANSFORM YOUR THINKING · TRANSFORM YOUR BODY · TRANSFORM YOUR LIFE

Date: ________________________   Day: M Tu W Th F Sa Su

Today's intention or Affirmation: ________________________________

Time	Hunger Rating Before	What did you eat?	What did you drink?	Satiety Rating After	Thinking	Feeling	Digestion	Mood

Hunger Level: From 1 to 5
Starving, Irritable, Strong urge to eat,
A little hungry, Starting to think about food

Satiety Level: From 6 to 10
Just starting to feel satisfied, Satisfied, very full, Uncomfortably full, Stuffed to the point of felling sick.

Mood: Did your mood change before, during or after eating? Did you feel better or worse? Happier, angrier, depressed, anxious, or upset after eating.

Understanding Food Labels

Although it is obvious certain foods like fruit, vegetables and whole grains are good for us, we are often left to make decisions about processed foods like cereal or frozen meals. Considering there are many manufacturers all making similar products, it is important to be able to identify what makes one product more nutritious or less caloric than another.

1

2

3a

3b

4

Nonfat Milk
Serving Size 8 fl oz (240mL)
Servings Per Container 2

Amount Per Serving

Calories 80   Calories from Fat 0

% Daily Value*

Total Fat 0g	0%
Saturated Fat 0g	0%
Cholesterol less than 5mg	1%
Sodium 130mg	5%
Total Carbohydrate 12g	4%
Dietary Fiber 0g	0%
Sugars 11g	
Protein 8g	

Vitamin A 8%   •   Vitamin C 4%

Calcium 30% • Iron 0% • Vitamin D 25%

* Percent Daily Values are based on a 2,000 calorie diet. Your daily values may be higher or lower depending on your calorie needs.

		Calories:	2,000	2,500
Total Fat	Less than		65g	80g
Sat Fat	Less than		20g	25g
Cholesterol	Less than		300mg	300mg
Sodium	Less than		2,400mg	2,400mg
Total Carbohydrate			300g	375g
Dietary Fiber			25g	30g

Section 1: The Serving Size

Looking at the serving size on the nutrition label is the first place to start. A serving size is listed in standardized units to make it easier to compare similar foods. The serving size allows you to know exactly how much you would need to consume all the calories and nutrients listed on the nutrition label. It is important to pay attention to the serving size and how many servings there are in the package. For example, in the sample food label, one serving is eight fluid ounces or one cup; however, if you drank the entire container, you would be consuming two servings, which would double all of the calories and other nutrient numbers.

Section 2: Calories

As we now know, calories are a measure of energy and can directly affect our weight. On the food label, the calories section lets us know how many calories there are in a single serving of that food product. For example, on this food label, one serving of milk is 80 calories. By drinking the entire container of milk, which is two servings, you would be consuming 160 calories.

Section 3: Nutrients
The nutrient section is divided into two parts. These sections lay out some key nutrients that can greatly impact your health and nutrition. 3a shows the macronutrients, cholesterol and sodium. The nutrients listed first (fat, cholesterol, and sodium) are what Americans tend to overeat and should be limited. Eating too much fat, saturated fat, trans fat (not shown), cholesterol and/or sodium can lead to certain chronic diseases such as heart disease, hypertension and obesity. The other nutrients in that section (carbohydrates and protein) simply allow you to see the macronutrient breakdown of the product. Currently, many Americans are trying to limit carbohydrates from the diet. However, carbohydrates are a necessary part of a balanced diet. Instead, it is a good idea to look at the sugars in a food. Sugars are listed as a subsection of carbohydrates.

3b shows us the nutrients that Americans tend to be lacking. Dietary fiber, listed above under carbohydrates, should be included in this list. In 3a we are given actual gram or milligram amounts, whereas in the 3b section we are only given percentages. These percentages will be addressed in section four.

Section 4: The Daily Values Footnote
The statement "Percent Daily Values are based on a 2,000-calorie diet" must be included on all food labels. However, the chart listed beneath the statement may not always be included depending on the size of the label. When the full footnote does appear, it will always be the same because it shows recommended dietary advice for all Americans and does not refer to a specific food item.

The percentages listed next to the nutrients indicate how much of the recommended daily allowance you would be consuming based on eating a 2,000-calorie diet. So for carbohydrates, you would be getting 4% of your recommended carbohydrate intake if you were consuming a 2,000 calorie diet. If you consume more calories, you will need even more carbohydrates in your diet.

Section 5: The Ingredient List (not shown)
The ingredient list is important to look at because it shows you exactly what is contained in the food product. It is especially important if you have any food allergies or intolerances. In addition, the ingredient list gives us an idea of how much of a certain ingredient is in a food product. The ingredients are listed in order of quantity used. So, if sugar is the first ingredient listed in a health food product, chances are that product is not too healthy.

MOVEMENT

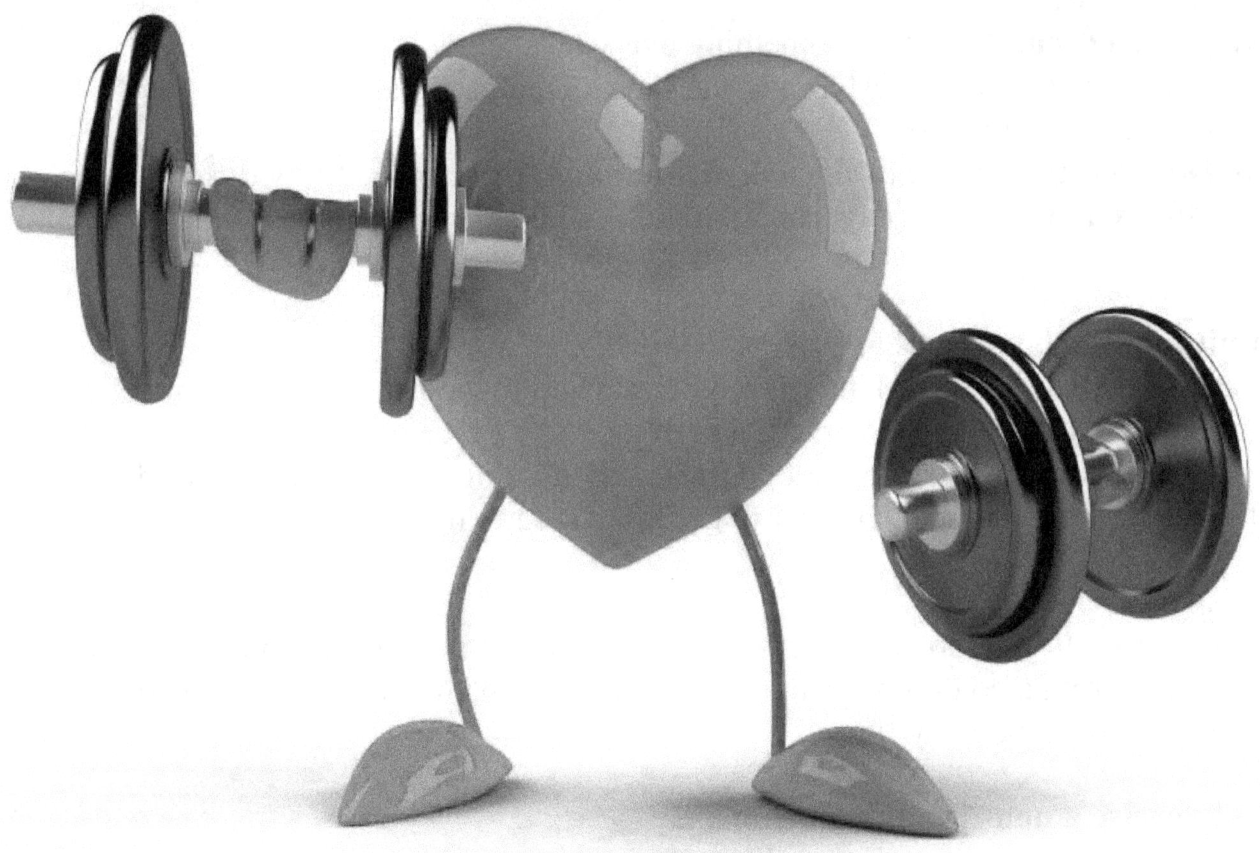

Movement Rules:

Life does not need to be complicated and neither does improving your lifestyle through improved health, increased fitness, and weight loss. Many people I have met struggle with exercising consistently. They have an improper or sour mindset about Fitness. Many believing that they must belong to a Fitness Center and do long, hard workouts every day to see results. Or they believe that while there, everybody knows what they are doing except for them. The good news is that better fitness can be achieved anywhere.

 Here are amazingly simple steps to take to look and feel great:

1. **MOVE TIMES 5**

   Move: Just Do Something
   Move More: Aim for a minimum of 100 minutes of 'Huffy Puffy' exercise every week
   Move More Often: Aim to do something everyday
   Move Quicker: Aim to go faster over the same distance or farther in the same amount of time
   Move Differently: Choose different activities or do the same activity differently (e.g. run or walk a different way, every day; run hills, flat, sand, slower for longer and shorter and quicker)

Put a dollar in a jar every time you work out, set a goal for yourself like $100.00 then use the money to treat yourself! Like a new outfit!

2. Commit to take the path of MOST resistance.
Escalators and elevators are a friend to weight gain and low performance. Remember Newton's law of motion – An object in motion stays in motion. An object at rest stays at rest. You are the object. If you begin your day moving, you will stay moving. If you begin your day with the habit of inactivity it is that much harder to get motivated to move.

3. Surprise Exercise.
Look for opportunities to move where you would not normally. Take a phone call while standing, pace during a conference call, set your laptop high so you can stand and work, take the furthest parking spot every time.

4. Make Exercise a non-negotiable priority.
We do what is important to us. Know that exercise/movement aids in reducing pains, increasing metabolism, creating sustained energy, and makes us feel better. **Do not accept not exercising.**

Fitness and Exercise Components:

1. **The Overload Principle**
2. **The FITT Principle**
3. **The Specificity Principle (S.A.I.D.)**
4. **The Rest and Recovery Principle**
5. **The Use or Lose Principle**

The Overload Principle

The Overload Principle is probably the most important principle of exercise and training. Simply stated, the Overload Principle means that the body will adapt to the workload placed upon it. The more you do, the more you will be capable of doing. This is how all the fitness improvements occur when exercising and training. When you stress the body through lifting a weight that the body is unaccustomed to lifting, the body will react by causing physiological changes in order to be able to handle that stress the next time it occurs. This concept is similar in cardiovascular training. If you ask the heart, lungs and endurance muscles to do work not previously done, it will make changes to the body to be able to handle that task better the next time. This is how people get stronger, bigger, faster and increase their physical fitness level.

When you are working out, you want to strive to somehow increase the workload you are doing above what you did on your previous workout, so you have overloaded your body to create a training adaptation. This increase in workout stress can be an exceedingly small increase, which over time will eventually be a significant increase or adaptation. To determine how to increase the workload of a given workout you need to understand the F.I.T.T Principle.

The F.I.T.T. Principle

An uncomplicated way to get started on developing a personal fitness program is utilizing the **F.I.T.T.** principle. This acronym stands for **Frequency**, **Intensity**, **Time,** and **Type**. These are the areas in which someone could increase or overload to improve physical fitness.

- **Frequency:** This refers to how often you will exercise. After any form of exercise is performed your body completes a process of rebuilding and repairing. So, determining the frequency of exercise is important to find a balance that provides just enough stress for the body to adapt and also allows enough rest time for healing.
- **Intensity:** Defined as the amount of effort or work that must be completed in a specific exercise. This too requires a good balance to ensure that the intensity is hard enough to overload the body but not so difficult that it results in over training, injury, or burnout.
- **Time:** Time is simply how long each individual session should last. This will vary based on the intensity and type.
- **Type:** What type of exercise will you be doing? Will an exercise session be primarily cardiovascular, resistance training or a combination of both? And what specific exercises will you perform.

Combining the Overload Principle and The F.I.T.T. Principle

	Resistance Training	Cardiovascular Training
Frequency	Increase the number of workout days	Increase the number of workout days
Intensity	Increase the resistance / weight	Increase pace or % of Max. Heart Rate
Time	Increase time involved in exercise or Increased repetitions.	Increase time involved in exercise
Type	Changing the exercise but still working the same area of the body	Changing the workout to a different cardio exercise. Ex. jogging to jump rope

Specific Adaptation to Imposed Demands
(S.A.I.D.) - The Specificity Principle

This principle is just how it sounds...how you exercise should be specific to your goals. If you are trying to improve your racing times, you should focus on speed workouts. If your main goal is simply health, fitness, and weight management, you should focus on total body strength, cardio, and a healthy diet. Make sure your training matches your goals. Regardless of the chosen goal, your body responds by adapting to any/all demands placed upon it.

The Rest and Recovery Principle

While we often focus on getting in as much exercise as possible, rest and recovery is also essential for reaching your weight loss and fitness goals. While you can often do cardio every day, though you may want to rest after very intense workouts, you should have at least a day of rest between strength training workouts. Make sure you do not work the same muscles two days in a row to give your body the time it needs to rest and recover.

The Eustress v Distress - "Use or Lose" Principle

The Principle of Use or Lose implies that when it comes to fitness, you "use it or lose it." This simply means that your muscles build strength (hypertrophy) with use and lose strength (atrophy) with lack of use. This also explains why we lose fitness when we stop exercising. Moving better requires several interconnected parts. Each of these is important to creating success in your exercise program.

- **Cardiovascular conditioning** - Your heart is the second most important organ, after the brain, and needs to be conditioned to achieve fitness success. The right cardio program can help you burn calories more efficiently while keeping you fit for increased activity.
- **Flexibility** - Your body needs to move efficiently. Overactive or underactive muscles can influence how you move, potentially leading to injuries. Therefore, you need to maintain proper posture and flexibility while you train.

 Innovation Fitness Solutions – Achievers Success Guide

- **Core Training** - Your core is made up of your abdominals, low back, and hips. It needs to be trained to keep you strong from the inside out and create better movement patterns for the arms and legs.
- **Balance Training** - Balance means being able to control your body during movement. In other words, training your body to control unwanted movement that might throw you off base helps you avoid falls and unwanted injuries throughout your life.
- **Resistance Training** - Keeping your body strong and increasing lean muscle mass are all integral to living a fit life. Resistance training is a key component of all of the above. The more muscle you have, the higher your metabolism, the lower your body fat percentage is, and the more you can do.

Each small working part has a role in overall fitness and must be trained accordingly. A healthy and fit lifestyle will encompass all the larger components as well as the smaller, moving parts.

Recovery - Optimize Your Sleep for Energy and Recovery

Sleep Recommendations:

- Learn the optimal hours you need to sleep. Everyone is different. Genetics determine how much sleep a person needs. The key is to determine how many hours you need to sleep each night to feel refreshed in the morning. Some people need 5, 6 or 8 hours a night. Most people know the number of hours that work best for them. Remember that number and set up your schedule to achieve those hours. This will allow your body to optimally function and prevent any sleep deficits.
- **Create a dark environment:** Less light triggers increased Melatonin release (your sleep hormone), which allows the body to enter a deeper quality of sleep.
- **Create a quiet environment:** Noisy environments have been shown to interrupt sleep cycles.
- **Sleep on a comfortable bed, pillow and sheets:** Comfort allows your muscles to relax and your body to stay in the proper alignment.
- **Sleep schedule:** Create a schedule that allows each day to be similar with wake time and bedtime. Keep the range plus or minus one hour.
- **Put your thoughts to bed. Write down all thoughts at least an hour before bed**: The mind seems to race at bedtime with thoughts of what to do the next day and life concerns. This happens to 90% of all clients we have worked with. The solution is making sure all thoughts are written down and dealt with at least one hour before bedtime.
- **Create proper down time:** Many people work, watch TV, or exercise before bedtime. The mind needs to be prepared for sleep.

Frequently Asked Questions

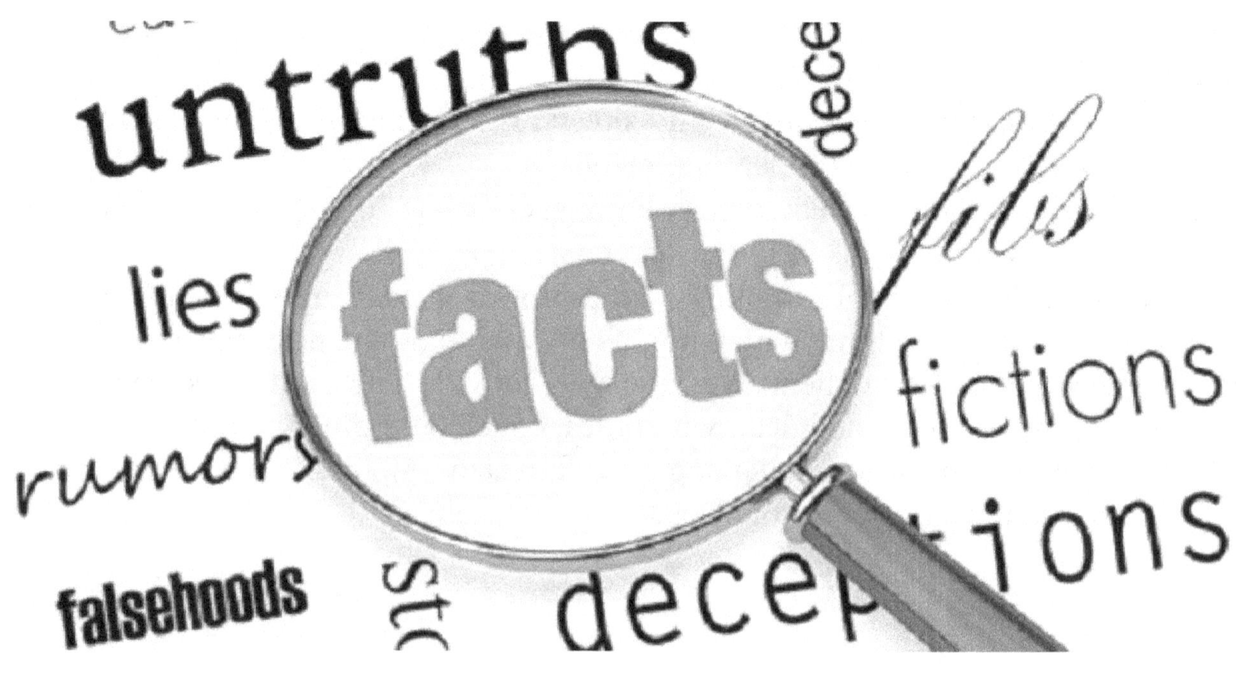

Question #1: "I'm new to this whole nutrition thing. Where do I start?"
Answer: Let us start by eliminating nutritional deficiencies.

This is always a fun one, because no one ever wants to believe they have nutritional deficiencies. Nutrition beginners do not need a major diet overhaul on day one. They do not need to "go Paleo" or "eliminate sugar".

- Your first step should be to open your eyes to the fact that you have one or more nutritional deficiencies (seriously, more than 80 percent of the population has at least one).
- Until nutritional deficiencies are removed, the body simply will not function properly and that makes any health or fitness goal a lot harder.

So, to eliminate deficiencies, your first order of business is to find workable strategies for rounding out the diet, so you get:

- A bit more protein
- Ample vitamins and minerals
- Sufficient healthy fats and
- More water

Once nutritional deficiencies are addressed, you can start to focus on things like food quality and portions. If you start to become impatient remind yourself that this process is not slow; it's systematic. It focuses on the things that are in your way right now. Once they are eliminated, progress happens fast.

Dietary Extremism
Then, Now and a Happy Medium

Then	Now	Happy Medium
Fats cause obesity and heart disease. Avoid fats at all costs.	There is no such thing as unhealthy fats or too much fat. Eat ALL the fat!	Fat intake should be based primarily on your personal preferences. Have mostly "healthy" fats (e.g. from nuts, olive oil, fatty fish, etc)
A healthy diet must be based primarily on carbs.	Carbs cause obesity and diabetes. Avoid carbs at all costs.	Have moderate amounts of carbs. If you are physically active and like carbs, have more of them.
Butter is extremely unhealthy. Cut it out altogether.	Not only is butter not unhealthy, but it's health-promoting. More is better. Put it in your coffee.	If you like butter, feel free to have some. In the context of an overall healthy diet, it's fine.
Breakfast is the most important meal of the day. You should always have breakfast.	Breakfast causes an insulin spike early in the day, making you fat and tired. Never have breakfast.	If you like having breakfast and it helps you better adhere to your diet, have breakfast.
You should eat every 2 hours or your metabolism will slow down.	You should fast for at least 16 hours every day. As with everything, more is better.	Adopt a meal frequency pattern that suits your lifestyle and helps you adhere to your diet.

The IFSism - The Ice-Sculpture
- Take your multi vitamin.
- Drink 32 oz more water daily.
- Take your Omega Fish Oils.
- Add Protein to at least 3 meals per day.

DO THIS FIRST. Try it for 30 days straight and let me know how you feel.

Question #2: "What's the best diet to follow?"
Answer: There is no "best diet".

As a highly experienced Coach, I get asked multiple time per day, "Which dietary "camp" do you belong to?" I maintain a neutral position on this. I consider myself to be a nutritional agnostic: someone who does not subscribe to any one dietary philosophy. Why? All dietary protocols have their pros and cons. What works best for one person will not work best for

 Innovation Fitness Solutions – Achievers Success Guide

another. Also, a diet that has worked best for someone in the past will not necessarily be what works best for them moving forward.

You need to do the detective work to find the approach to eating that works best for you right now, whether it be Paleo or vegan, high-carb or low-carb, tight budget or unlimited funds or some blend of all of these. The truth is, the human body is amazingly adaptable to a vast array of diets, so the best diet is the one that:

- Matches your unique physiology,
- Includes foods that you enjoy enough to follow consistently, and
- Is realistic for them in terms of life logistics and budget.

I can make people lean, strong, and healthy on a plant-based or a meat-based diet. I can help improve their health with organic, free-range foods and with conventional foods. You can lose weight on a low food budget or an unlimited one. It just takes a little know-how and a system for using the best practices across all diets.

Question #3: "Is counting calories important for weight loss?"
Answer: While it feels logical, counting calories is often complex, time consuming, and full of errors. The good news: There is a better way.

Weight management is a simple equation: Eat more than you burn, and you gain weight. Eat less and you lose weight.

But the physiology behind "calories in, calories out" is much more complex and dynamic than most people realize. Plus, it is highly imprecise. Studies estimate that there is typically an error of up to 25 percent on the 'calories in' side, and on the 'calories out' side. That can be anywhere from a 25% - 50% error. Beyond that, counting calories is an external system (outside of your body). Those who count calories are less likely to see lasting results because they are outsourcing appetite awareness to the food-label gods. To really win at calorie control, tuning in to your internal hunger signals and creating internal systems are vital components of success.

For these reasons, and more, for most people, counting calories is a lot of work for extraordinarily little benefit. Instead of calorie counting, we recommend two primary things –
1. Nutritional Targets (see page 69).
2. A hand-measure system for portion sizes (which we have already discussed).

This system counts your calories for you, and gets your macronutrients lined up, without having to do any annoying food-label math. Plus, your hands are portable, they go wherever you go (unless you are Luke Skywalker), making portion sizing very convenient. In addition, your hands are generally scaled to your size the bigger you are, the bigger your hands, so the more food you need and the more food you get.

Question #4: "Should I avoid carbs?"
Answer: No but let us make sure you're getting the right kind of carbs.

Ask almost any client what they need to do to lose a few pounds and they will probably say, "Cut back on carbs." However, most of us would do best eating a moderate amount of quality carbs; whole grains (when tolerated), fruit, potatoes, sweet potatoes, beans, and legumes, etc. We emphasize **moderate**, of course.
- For men, this usually means about 1-2 cupped handfuls per meal
- And women, about ½-1 cupped handful per meal.

Bottom line: carbs are *not* inherently fattening, especially whole food sources. And getting adequate carbs can help you exercise harder and recover better, optimizing progress.
Yep, this is a controversial position to take, but it works. And while avoiding carbs may facilitate rapid weight loss initially, it is not practical, or necessary, for long-term success.

IFS Food Rules
- Avoid "Cardboard carbs".
- Choose "greenface".
- Veggies and berries are your friend.
- The more you work out and the higher the intensity, the more carbs you need.
- Cutting Carbs causes rapid initial weight loss (due to water loss) and will nearly ALWAYS backfire.

Question #5: Are all calories equal?
Answer: The people who like to use this slogan that "a calorie isn't a calorie" usually do so because
1. Some foods are more nutrient dense than others and
2. Different nutrient profiles impact the **thermic effect of food** - a term used to describe the energy expended by our bodies in order to consume (bite, chew, and swallow) and process (digest, transport, metabolize, and store) food - in different ways.

Although both points are true, that explanation still does not make valid the claim that a calorie is not a calorie. To understand why it does not, we must first establish what a calorie is.
- A calorie is a unit of energy equal to the amount of heat needed to raise the temperature of 1 gram of water by 1 °C. In short, a calorie is a unit of heat.

With this definition in mind, for it to be accurate that a "calorie isn't a calorie," some type of food would have to provide calories that aren't a unit of energy equal to the amount of heat needed to raise the temperature of 1 gram of water by 1 °C. So, name a food that provides calories, whether it be a nutrient-poor or nutrient-dense food, that are not a unit of heat. The fact that you cannot name a food (because there are not any) proves that a calorie is a calorie because all calories are units of heat.

This highlights the fundamental problem with the justification that is often given for saying that a calorie is not a calorie. The problem is that it conflates a nutrient makeup of the food with its energy-producing value. So, this certainly is not just semantics, it's why we have terms like "nutrient-poor (EDNP) foods" and "nutrient-dense foods" to delineate the nutrient makeup of the food from its energy-producing value.

Conflation is the logical fallacy of treating two, or more, distinct subjects (that may be related or similar to the other) as if they were one, which obscures analysis of the distinctions between the two concepts and, therefore produces errors or misunderstandings. And we see both errors from fitness and nutrition "experts" who say this and misunderstanding from their clients and followers who they're saying it to.

The people who use the slogan "a calorie isn't a calorie" are making an error when they bring up nutritional values and the thermic effect of food (TEF) when talking about what they're claiming is and isn't a calorie. This is because what makes a calorie a calorie by definition, as we established above, has nothing to do with nutrient profiling or the thermic effect of food -- it is simply an *energy value*. That is it!

The major misunderstanding people often get from the slogan "a calorie is not a calorie" is that it implies that caloric quantity is not a crucial factor for one to consider, as one need only to pay attention to the quality (i.e., nutrient density) of the foods they eat. However, as I established above, both food quality and quantity are key factors that should be considered together, because, as important as it is to eat high quality, nutrient-dense foods for general health, you can still gain fat from eating "healthy" if you eat too many calories relative to what you're burning.

Question #6: "Should I avoid grains?"
Answer: No, most people trying to stay lean do best with a reasonable amount of whole grains.

Grain discussions are trendy right now, as many people have suggested they're dietary enemy #1 and should be eliminated, other camps label sugar as enemy #1 and yet, others label fats as the worst cause of weight gain and poor health. This is hot news as, just ten years ago; grains were supposedly one of the healthiest foods on the planet. From our perspective, grains are not as evil as they have been made out to be by the Paleo and Whole30 camps. At the same time, they are not the superfood vegans and macrobiotic eaters suggest either. As is usual, instead of the black or white, good, or bad view, we teach the shades of grey.

Bottom line
While you do not need to eat grains, unless you have celiac disease or a FODMAP intolerance, there is absolutely no need to avoid them. Most people follow a better, more health-promoting diet if they are allowed grains in reasonable amounts, along with a wide array of other non-grain carb sources like fruit, potatoes, sweet potatoes, beans, lentils, etc.

Remember, it is the ability to follow a diet consistently over time that provides the greatest results, regardless of what that diet is. And unless you are intolerant, there's no good reason to totally exclude certain foods, especially foods you enjoy.

Question #7: "If I eat well for x # of days, is it ok to have a treat meal or a day that I am not so "strict"?"
Answer: Cutting out favorite foods completely is a bad idea. But cutting back?
Cut back on the frequency of cheat foods without depriving yourself a "treat" now and then. You will notice it's much easier to stick with your diet than battering yourself over a restricted diet. The truth is that moderation is not cheating, it's part of a well-designed plan, it's setting yourself up for success in the long-term, and it's perfectly acceptable. Many people are convinced that they must follow the "All or None" approach to eating (i.e.: "I am on a diet, so I cannot have bad, unhealthy, high calorie foods"). This approach repeated over many years causes a start and stop style rather than a fluid continuum.

Question #8: "What are some eating strategies to help with weight loss?"
Answer: Before we discuss eating strategies, I find that it is vital to have your mindset on what goal you are pursuing. I find that when people state, "weight loss" they truly mean "fat loss". However, you must make a clear distinction between the two, because if your goal is truly weight loss, then any eating style or diet will do if it creates and energy deficit. You have heard "eat less, move more" over and over. For weight loss, this physiological principle is true. This is important because weight loss is arbitrary and can include weight that you did not intend or desire to lose (water, muscle). Fat Loss programming must follow a more specific protocol than weight loss.

Eating better for health and fat loss begins with FOCUS. Try these tips for 30 days and feel the difference in your energy, vitality, strength and focus. Incorporate them for life and watch who you can become! There are no tricks, just consistent application of proven fundamentals. Stick to the basics, be consistent and become healthy and fit!

FOOD: Energy In
- Begin planning meals with choosing Protein and Veggies first. Strive to eat these at every meal.
- Increase water by drinking up to eight, 8oz. glasses of water a day. Strive for an intake of 1 oz/lb of BW.
- Think "Subtraction by Addition". What can you ADD to your food intake (Proteins, Veggies, Fruits, Grains) not what do you need to take away? **Bonus:** Eating Calorically sparse / Nutritionally Dense foods will increase fullness and provide greater nutrition.
  - Decrease saturated and trans fats by limiting processed, fried and fatty foods.
  - Increase fiber by choosing complex carbohydrates as well as fruits and vegetables.
  - Eat four or five small meals three to four hours apart to help prevent hunger.
- Moderate sodium intake to help prevent water retention and bloating.
- Eat slowly to help prevent overeating.

- Stay clear of the PERFECTIONIST mindset. One meal or unhealthy food choice will not doom you. Your habits make or break your success.

Question #9: "How can I minimize stomach discomfort (bloating, distention, gas) following a meal?"
Answer:
1. Chew your food – (SOE, Speed of Eating)
2. Do not preload the fork
3. Drink water consistently
4. Consistent sodium intake
5. Control meal volume and calories

Question #10: "What (and when) should I eat around my workouts?"
Answer: It depends on your goals. Let us talk about those… then we can come up with specific recommendations for you.

Contrary to popular media, **most people are best served by eating excellent quality whole foods in reasonable amounts**, without having to focus on specific workout nutrition products or protocols. Eat a normal, balanced meal 1-2 hours before and after exercise. This will provide adequate protein and carbs to both fuel the workout and maximize recovery/adaption.

A few options for this for those of us on the run
1. PB & J on wheat bread
2. Greek Yogurt (no sugar added)
3. A piece of fruit and a whole fat cheese stick

The DONT's of Workout Nutrition
- **Do not overeat**. You will feel lethargic due to most of your energy going toward digestive processes.
- **Do not NOT eat**. You can occasionally get away with not eating for a cardio workout (as fat is the primary fuel source). However, this is not the case for Strength Training. The fuel source for this activity is **Glycogen**, which is supplied by Carbohydrates. Carbs are consistently required to be replenished every few hours.
- **Do not try to "outsmart" your body**. It does not matter what you want to happen, the processes and energy requirements in Physiology happen no matter what.
- **Do not skip your meal because you feel like you ate too much already**. This may be true but will not help you to maximize your workouts. Have a small meal or snack and get back on track.
- **Do not think "I need to burn fat during my workout."** This sounds counter-intuitive, but Fat Loss is a *result*, not a goal. This happens from consistent energy deficits and proper nutrition. A goal of training is to aid the body in building muscle and burning calories, which will eventually come from fat but not during your workouts.

Question #11: "Should I drink less alcohol?"
Answer: If optimal health and fitness is your priority, consider reevaluating your drinking habits.

You may balk at that answer initially, but once I lay out the facts and make it clear that *I am not telling you not to drink*, your ears will open. There is a lot of confusion about whether drinking is good for you or not. That is mainly because the news media likes to play up new studies revealing the possible cardiovascular benefits of alcohol. But the truth is, no one *really* knows who will benefit from light to moderate alcohol consumption. Meanwhile, any level of drinking, even "moderate", comes with health risks that should be considered.

It is called The French Paradox. In theory, if we abide by the recommendations of 1 drink per day for women and 2 drinks a day for men, it lowers our LDL (bad cholesterol) and increases our HDL (good cholesterol). Exceeding these recommendations will result in the **OPPOSITE** effect and "worsen" our health. Heavy drinking (more than 7 drinks a week for women and more than 14 per week for men) increases the risk for a long list of health problems involving the heart, brain, immunity, hormones, liver, and metabolism.

But even light to moderate drinking can affect sleep, appetite, and decision making, which absolutely can have a negative impact on your health and fitness goals. Still, drinking is an undeniable part of culture, and when enjoyed reasonably, it can be delicious and fun.

I'm going to help you sort out your priorities to determine the best level of drinking for you. Next, I encourage you to **track your drinking habits**, and how your drinking habits make you feel physically and psychologically, for a couple weeks. Most drinkers consume a lot more alcohol than they think, and when they stop to evaluate, many decide that it would feel better to cut back.

Question #12: "Does the Paleo Diet live up to the hype?"
Answer: Mostly, yes. But not for the reasons you think.

The Paleo Diet is one of the most popular nutrition approaches in the world right now. There is no doubt that it works for many people. However, the reason it works has little to do with the story the Paleo proponents tell (evolutionary adaptation, inflammation, etc.). Paleo does work for a lot of people because it emphasizes mostly whole-food sources of lean protein, vegetables, fruits, and healthy fats.

Paleo is starting to incorporate more high-quality carbs, grass-fed dairy, red wine, and other things that used to be "off limits", but the diet can still be too restrictive for some folks. In the end, Paleo likely gets more right than wrong. And if you want to follow it, you can do it in a sane, reasonable, and sustainable manner. But for most, it is unnecessary to follow such a strict dietary ideology. You can take the good from the Paleo approach and get rid of the silly dogma.

Question #13: "Should I do a detox or juice cleanse?"
Answer: Probably not. Most popular detox diets do not remove toxins or lead to fat loss.

Lots of people are worried about the effect of modern lifestyle factors like poor nutrition, sleep deprivation, stress, and environmental pollutants on their health. Detox diets and juice cleanses, which have come into vogue as an efficient way to "supposedly" lose weight and rid the body of impurities do not clean out toxins or help you lose body fat. In fact, detox diets can work *against* these goals by bypassing the body's natural detoxification systems and creating a feast-or-famine cycle of eating.

Among many problems, detoxes and cleanses often:
- Are protein deficient
- Are extremely low in energy
- Cause unhealthy blood-sugar swings
- Cause GI tract dysfunction and
- Lead to a yoyo of restrictive eating and overcompensation.

If doing a juice cleanse or detox diet helps you get ready to make further helpful and sustainable changes in your life, OK. I would caution and monitor your protocol. However, we prefer **helping you build life-long skills and incorporate daily practices** to improve your health, performance, body composition and your bodies normal detoxification system, without extreme, and unsustainable, things like detoxes and cleanses.

Question #14: "How can I improve my sleep and stress management?"
Answer: The answer is unique to every person. Sleep is just as important as nutrition and exercise when it comes to improving your health, performance, and body composition.

To achieve these goals, you should focus on:
- Creating a sleep routine, including having a regular schedule.
- Limiting alcohol and caffeine, especially in the afternoon/evening.
- Choosing de-stressing activities before bed.
- Setting an appropriate room temperature for sleep.
- Making the room dark.
- Keeping the room quiet.
- Waking up appropriately, with light exposure and soft noise.

As for stress, it's all about finding the sweet spot. Too much stress, or the wrong kind, can harm our health. Yet stress can also be a positive force in our lives, keeping us focused, alert, and at the top of our game. It all depends on what kind of stress it is, how prepared we are to meet it and how we view it. Since stress affects the mind, body, and behavior in many ways, **everyone experiences stress differently**. Each of us has a unique "recovery zone," whether it is physical or psychological, and our recovery zone depends on several factors. It is critical to understand these strategies and skills to view and handle your own stress load appropriately.

 Innovation Fitness Solutions – Achievers Success Guide

The following can increase stress tolerance or diminish stress load:
- Meditation or yoga
- Outdoor time
- Snuggling a pet
- Listening to relaxing music
- Deep breathing

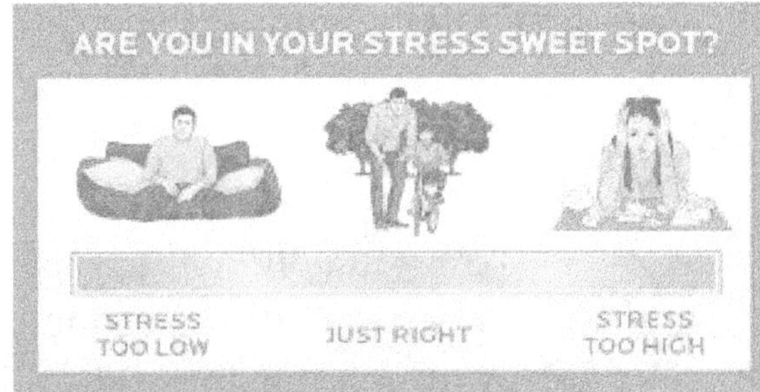

Question #15: "How can I react positively to stress?"
Answer: The first step to reacting to stress in a positive way is to understand that stress is a natural part of life. Meaning, you have got to know that avoidance of stress is highly unlikely. However, being better prepared for stressors, having a plan in place to identify when you are feeling stressed, and having skills and tools at the ready will mentally prepare you to better handle stress and stressful situations. **A few of these tools -**

1. **Mindfulness/awareness -** Being present and aware of how you are thinking and how you are feeling is vital to a positive outcome. Practice "checking in" with yourself when you are in a clear mind. Ask yourself questions such as: How am I feeling? Am I tense? Am I having recurring focus on one challenge or problem? Am I in an even mood or am I becoming short in my temper? A consistent "check-in" will better keep you on track and aware of your feelings.
2. **Breathe -** You can either focus on a problem or you can focus on a solution. One way in which you can focus on a solution is to slow down and breathe. Find a quiet spot where you can be alone for 3-5 minutes. Breathe in deeply through your nose and out through your mouth. Repeat.
3. **Develop a "mantra" -** A mantra is a saying that is simple and repeatable. It will be your go-to phrase to keep you focused on what you want. An example of a positive and simple mantra is, "I am strong enough to face any challenge" or "I get to choose my mood and my reactions."
4. **Maintain Perspective -** Focus on Big Picture things. Ask yourself if what you are getting upset about will matter in an hour, or tomorrow. In most cases it will not. This perspective shift will allow you to maintain focus on what matters rather than spending time being upset over trivial things.
5. **Avoid Perfectionism -** As a part of humanity, we are prone to mistakes. Remember this. No one handles everything perfectly. If we can "live and learn," then we are on the right track. Gain lessons and tools from your mistakes to enable you to not get so stressed and rebound from stress quicker.

The Hunger Scale

1	2	3	4	5	6	7	8	9	10
Starving and feeling weak/dizzy.	Very hungry, irritable, low energy, large amounts of stomach growling.	Pretty hungry, stomach is beginning to growl.	Beginning to feel hungry.	Satisfied, niether hungry nor full.	Slightly full/ pleasantly full.	Slightly uncomfortable.	Feeling Stuffed.	Very uncomfortable, stomach aches.	So full you feel sick.

Question 16 - How can I reduce or minimize hunger and cravings?
Differentiate between hunger (needs) and appetite (wants/habits).

Hunger
Check your *water intake*.
- Are you achieving at least 96 oz per day?
- When was the last time you drank before feeling hungry?
- Add in the habit of drinking before you eat or setting an alarm to remind you to drink.
- Check your *food quality*
  - Complex foods such as vegetables, lean proteins, whole grains and fruit have a satiating (keep you full longer) effect.
- Check your meal amounts (Quantity)
  - Are you eating enough food volume to sustain you to your next meal?
  - Are your meals macro-nutrient balanced?
- Check your food structure (combinations)
  - Are you eating Protein at every meal?
  - Are you eating enough fat?
- Check your food timing
  - Are your meals frequent enough to stave off hunger and cravings?

Summary
Understand that stress is natural and with practice you can maintain control of your mood by being prepared for impending stressors. Smile, breathe and stay happy!

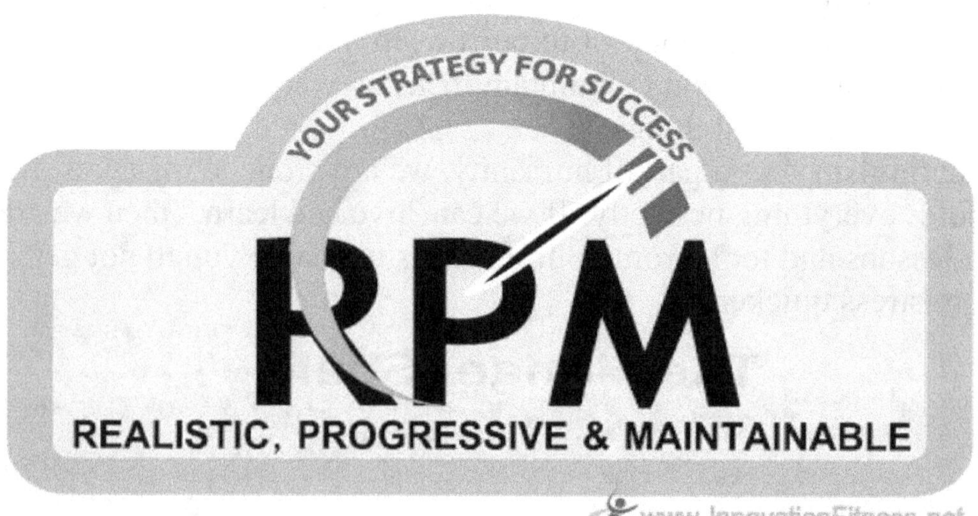

1. **How much cardiovascular and weight/ resistance training should I be doing weekly?**

The answer to this question is completely dependent on your goal.

- Most athletes will need to do at least 4-5 days weekly of weight training and cardiovascular work plus sports specific practice and training.
- For most novice fat loss clients, it is much less. Two to three days weekly should be sufficient when you begin a Fat Loss plan.

Keep in mind that we are implementing strategies for Food Intake and Energy Expenditure. There is no need to rely on excessive cardio exercise.

2. **What is the best cardiovascular exercise to lose weight?**

The simple answer is anything that you will enjoy doing. Innovation Fitness utilizes H.I.I.T in our sessions and most of our Group Training sessions have a cardiovascular component built into the sessions. Many exercise participants create undue stress for themselves trying to find the "magic exercise" that burns the most calories in the shortest period. The reality is that this is only a short-term solution. Your body is incredibly adaptive, which requires you to change your workout, both Cardio and Resistance, on a regular basis.

I suggest starting with the exercise that you enjoy the most and manipulate the intensity for 3-4 weeks. At that point, you will be ready to change your mode and force the body to start adjusting to something new. This will keep you burning the most calories in every workout.

3. **How many repetitions are best when weight training for weight loss?**

The goal of resistance training while in a fat loss plan is to burn the most calories in the least amount of time and to increase tonicity (muscle hardness/definition). The repetition range should be altered based on how long you have been doing the same type of program.

Remember: your body *adapts* to all new stimuli. The more frequent the stimulus, the quicker the body adapts. It is important to make changes to your exercise type, repetition range, weight lifted and exercise order frequently.

4. **How many calories will I burn, on average, during a one-hour workout?**

Based on the research done by the National Institute on Health and the Taylor Code (an estimate of energy expenditure during exercise), you can burn between 300-600 calories per hour during resistance training and 200-500 calories per hour during cardio exercise. If your goal is to increase calorie expenditure during exercise, it is essential that you keep your exercise program fresh and new. Making changes to your exercises, exercise order, sets, reps or amount of weight lifted will spark the body to burn more calories during and after the workout

There are multiple factors that will change this estimate:

- Body Weight, Conditioning, Intensity of Movement, Frequency of the stimulus.

5. **When doing a workout that combines both cardio and weight resistance training, is it more beneficial to do weights first and then cardio or vice versa? Why?**

Recent research from the nationally accredited personal training certifications recommends an exercise order as follows:

- Cardio Warm-up, Dynamic Warm-Up/ Stretching, Resistance Training, Flexibility, Cardio Exercise, Cool Down.

However, if you are crunched for time and/or get bored doing resistance training prior to cardio, don't fret; movement, no matter what order, will always be beneficial to calorie burning and improving health over not moving.

For fat loss, the goal is to maintain tone and increase caloric burn during the workout. With that in mind, the exercise order is not nearly as important for an event athlete. For specific athletic events, this will also change depending on the goal. An individual who is a strength athlete will be best suited to do a warm-up followed by resistance training than cardio. An athlete who is specific to endurance that utilizes resistance training for strength purposes will be better off focusing on their specific sport needs first.

6. How should I measure my success?

There are multiple ways to measure success. The physical methods will be your bodyweight, your body fat percentage, how your clothes are fitting and your ability to perform your workout activities and activities of daily living better and more efficiently.

The psychological measures will be how much better and more confident you are feeling about yourself. The improvements to your self-esteem and your quality of life are endless when proper eating and exercise become a part of your life. I also strongly urge you to take Before and After photos, which can be an extremely beneficial way to provide positive feedback. The day-to-day changes are incrementally small but when seen over the course of 1, 2 or more months, the visual aid can be staggering.

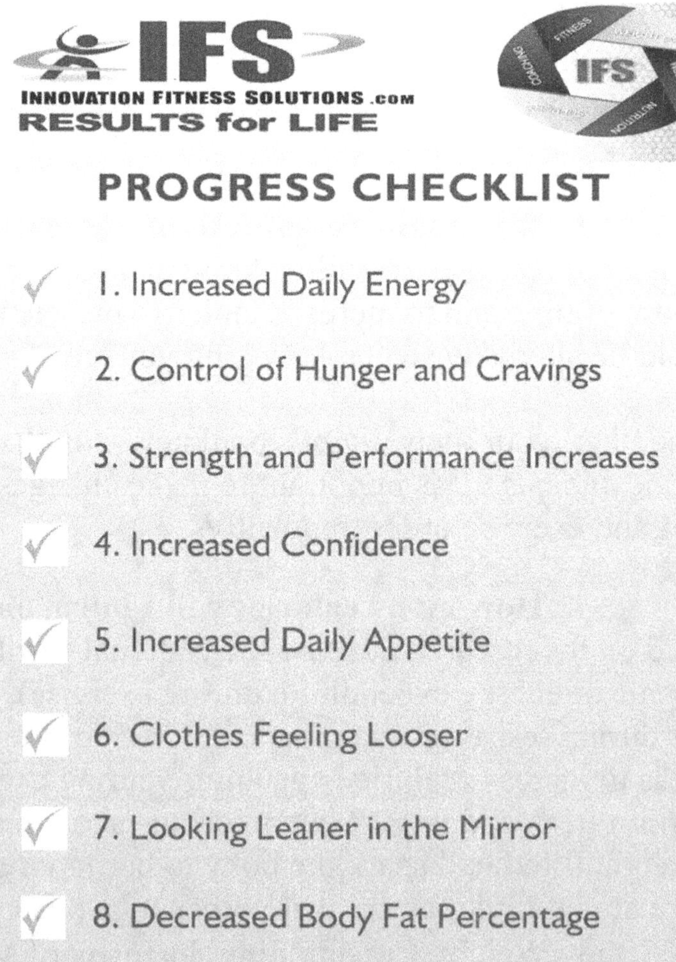

Reality Check – Myth Busting

Myth #1: You Can Target One Area of Your Body for Weight Loss (AKA: Spot Reduction)

Reality: The muscle does not "OWN" the fat that surrounds it. This is a myth, pure and simple. No matter how much exercise you do for a specific region of the body, it is physically impossible to lose body fat in a targeted area. Worse yet, the areas of your body that gain fat the fastest are the last to see it go. Fat is gained or lost throughout the entire the body. But do not despair. Just because you are not losing fat from exactly where you want to does not mean you will not lose it from there eventually. It will just take a bit longer. Stay consistent.

You don't get to choose where the fat goes on, why do you think you get to choose where it comes off? - You can't target fat loss.

Myth #2: Lifting Weights Can Make You Look Bulky.

Reality: This is a myth that deters many women from strength training. In fact, what determines the amount of muscle bulk a person has is largely dependent on genetic factors. Therefore, for the typical woman, and man, the chances of looking like Arnold Schwarzenegger are very slim. Weight training is also an important part of any exercise plan, according to the American Heart Association web site; while aerobic activities help your heart and lungs and stretching improves your flexibility, weight training will improve your strength and endurance, and a combination of all three makes for an optimal exercise plan. Weight training also burns significant calories over many other forms of exercise.

Myth #3: Avoid Fats.

Reality: Fats increase your sense of fullness. Fat has more calories per gram than protein and carbohydrate so cutting back on fat will help you to reduce calories. However, you do not want to avoid fat completely. Your brain and heart require fats to function. Studies show that fat contributes to a sense of satiety and adds flavor to many foods. Eliminating fat from your diet will increase your hunger. Avoid saturated and trans fats found in meat, poultry skin, high-fat dairy, eggs, processed baked goods and fried foods. Instead, choose monounsaturated and polyunsaturated fats found in fish, nuts, and vegetable oils (e.g., olive oil, canola oil, peanut oil).

Myth #4: Never Eat After 8 PM.

Fact: Calories do not own watches. The important thing is to focus on *how many* calories you consume throughout the day; not *when* you eat them. Many people intentionally save 200 to 300 calories to eat at night. Sure, eating a big meal before you go to bed may give you some indigestion, but it will not necessarily result in weight gain. Eating at night may be the best time for you. You are at home, the kids are in bed, and you have time to enjoy your food. Bottom line, it is possible to have a late snack or meal and stick to your diet plan.

Myth #5: If You Eat Well, You Do Not Need to Supplement Your Diet with a Multivitamin.
Reality: Nobody eats perfectly 365 days of the year.
Regardless of whether you eat well or not, it is very difficult to consume all of the necessary vitamins and minerals on a daily basis, especially if you are following a low calorie diet. Consuming the recommended amounts of all vitamins and minerals allows you to maximize exercise performance, body fat reduction, lean tissue development and your health. If your body is deficient in inadequacies, any nutrient, the body will break down muscle tissue to release more nutrients. As a result, your metabolism may slow down slightly due to a reduction in muscle mass. Supplementing with a daily multivitamin also allows you to compensate for any nutritional inadequacies.

Myth #6: Doing cardio first thing in the morning on an empty stomach is the best way to lose fat. What do you think?
Reality: Well, it is a way, but not necessarily the best way.
When you awaken, your body is in a fasting metabolic state and burning fewer calories per unit of time than usual. Consuming some food will perk your metabolic rate up (hence, the term "breakfast" – breaking the fast). Additionally, glycogen stores are depleted by as much as 80%. This will adversely affect your ability to workout at a high intensity and may cause weakness, dizziness, and lead to early fatigue. If meal preparation time is an issue, the use of a meal replacement drink can be helpful. The theory behind fasted cardio is that you rely on fat for fuel because you have no other sources of energy. What is going to happen when you replenish your stores? It will most likely be stored as fat.

Myth #7: Protein is bad for your bones and kidneys

Carbs and fats often take the blame for various health issues, but the third macronutrient is not always spared by the media. Protein has often been accused of causing bone and kidney damage.

Let us tackle those two claims one at a time. More protein in the diet has been linked to more calcium in the urine. Two reasons have been suggested to explain this phenomenon: Your body draws from its calcium stores (in bones) to buffer the acid load caused by dietary protein. This has led researchers to suggest that higher protein intake could cause greater bone loss Most studies that looked at protein intake and calcium excretion list dairy products as a protein source, so higher urinary calcium could simply be the result of higher calcium intake (i.e., more calcium in, more calcium out). Therefore, looking only at calcium *excretion* was not enough. Subsequent studies showed that dietary protein promotes dietary-calcium absorption and that high protein intake "promotes bone growth and retards bone loss whereas low-protein diet is associated with higher risk of hip fractures." All in all, current evidence suggests that **protein actually has a neutral or even protective effect on bones.**

Other studies determined that high protein diets increased *glomerular filtration rate* (GFR), a marker for waste filtration in the kidneys. It was argued that increased GFR was a sign that undue stress was put on the kidneys,] but later research has shown that kidney damage does not occur as a result of diets high in protein.

In conclusion, randomized trials thus far have not shown high protein diets to have harmful effects on the bones or kidneys in otherwise healthy adults.[9]

The Truth: Protein, even in large amounts, is not harmful to your bones or kidneys (unless you suffer from a pre-existing condition).

Myth #8 Carbs are bad for you

For decades, fat was the enemy; today, there is a new scapegoat: *carbs*. Vilifying carbs and insulin seem to get more popular by the year.

Many people believe that the popular glycemic index and the lesser-known insulin index rank foods by their "unhealthiness". Yet, available research on low-glycemic diets have seen results ranging from neutral to modest improvements even for diabetics. Furthermore, a low-glycemic diet doesn't universally perform better than other diet patterns.]

Similarly, the carbohydrate-insulin model of obesity, which theorizes that obesity is caused by carbs and the insulin response they evoke, is not well-supported by the evidence In 2017, a meta-analysis of 32 controlled feeding studies was published. Some of those studies were metabolic ward studies and some were free-living studies, but in each case, meals were provided by the researchers, who wished to ensure that each diet would provide specific amounts of calories and nutrients (within each study, the diets were equal in calories and protein but not in fat and carbs). So, what were the results? These studies help us understand the mechanism of weight loss, more so than a diets real-world effectiveness. Low-fat diets resulted in greater fat loss (by an average of 16 grams per day) and greater energy expenditure (by an average of 26 Calories per day). This would give low-fat diets a fat-loss advantage, though one "so small as to be physiologically meaningless".

These results are consistent with long-term free-living studies of low-carb or keto diets that test a diets real-world effectiveness. Meta-analyses of RCTs of show that neither provide clinically relevant weight loss differences when compared to higher-carb diets.

Cutting down carb intake (especially processed carbs) can be helpful if it helps you eat healthier. But if cutting carbs makes you eat worse or feel worse or you cannot stick with it, you should consider other options. If you wish to lose weight, what matters is not to replace fat by carbs or carbs by fat, but to end most days on a caloric deficit.

The Truth: If you do not overindulge, there is nothing inherently harmful about carbohydrates.

Myth #8 Egg yolks are bad for you

If there is one thing the media is good at, it's scaring you away from perfectly healthy foods. Eggs have been demonized because their yolks, which are chock-full of nutrients, contain high levels of cholesterol. Yet, for most people, eating foods high in cholesterol is not strongly linked to an increase in blood cholesterol levels. More to the point, in clinical trials, no association was found between eggs and cardiovascular disease, except *maybe* in some people with specific pre-existing conditions such as diabetes or hyperglycemia.PMID|23676423

The Truth: Eggs are a great source of protein, fats, and other nutrients. Their association with high

Myth #9 Red meat is bad for you

The common refrain: red meat causes cancer.

Absolute statements are why we have so many nutrition myths. Cancer is particularly difficult to discuss in absolutes. After all, almost everything we eat has the potential to be involved in cancer development Yet, red meat has been fingered as a likely culprit.

Some compounds — such as *polyaromatic hydrocarbons* (PAHs), found in smoked meats — have been found to damage the genome, which is the first step to potential cancer. Current evidence suggests that processed red meats, particularly those that are more charred during cooking, *can* pose a greater cancer risk for people with poor diets and lifestyles. But if you moderate your red meat intake, exercise regularly, eat your fruits and veggies, consume adequate fiber, don't smoke, and drink only in moderation, red meat's effect on cancer isn't something to worry too much about.

The Truth: Fears about red meat causing cancer are vastly exaggerated. Making healthy lifestyle choices (such as staying at a healthy weight, exercising, and not smoking) is more important than micromanaging your red meat intake. Still, if you plan to decrease your intake of red meat, start with the kind that has been cured, smoked, or highly processed.

Myth #10 Salt is bad for you

Some myths contain a grain of truth. Studies have associated excess salt with hypertension (high blood pressure), kidney damage,[1] and an increased risk of cognitive decline.

But salt (sodium) is an essential mineral; its consumption is critical to your health. The problem is when you consume too much sodium and too little potassium.

Another issue is the source of all that salt. The average North American eats an incredible amount of salty processed foods[1] — which means that people who consume a lot of salt tend to consume a lot of foods that are generally unhealthy. That makes it hard to tease apart sodium's effects from overall dietary effects. Except for individuals with salt-sensitive hypertension, the evidence in support of low sodium intakes is less conclusive than most people would imagine. As it stands, both exceedingly high *and very low* intakes are associated with cardiovascular disease.

The Truth: Salt reduction is important for people with salt-sensitive hypertension, and excess salt intake is associated with harm. But drastically lowering salt intake has not shown uniform benefit in clinical trials. Most people will benefit more from a diet of mostly unprocessed foods than they would from micromanaging their salt intake.

Myth #11 Bread is bad for everyone

Bread has taken a beating over the past few years (especially white bread). The bread detractors generally make two arguments against its consumption:

1. Bread will make you fat.

2. Bread contains lots of **gluten**, which is bad for you.

Bread will not inherently make you fat, but it tends to be dense in calories and therefore easy to overeat. And of course, most people will eat bread with other high-calorie foods, such as butter, peanut butter, jam, or honey. This can lead to a caloric surplus and thus to weight gain over time. Moreover, while bread can be *part* of a healthful diet, a bread-centric diet can crowd out more nutrient-rich foods, notably fruits and vegetables.

Also, some people choose to avoid bread entirely because of its gluten content. Gluten critics claim that any amount of gluten (a protein, ironically, not a carb) is a danger to all. While "all" is an exaggeration, it is indeed possible to suffer from non-celiac gluten sensitivity. However, it is also possible for your wheat sensitivity to be caused by other compounds, such as FODMAPS (short-chain carbohydrates known to promote intestinal distress by fermenting and producing gas).

White bread vs. whole-wheat bread

You may have heard that eating bread is all right if it's whole-wheat bread. While white bread (made from wheat flour) and whole-wheat bread provide a similar number of calories, whole-wheat bread has a lower glycemic index and insulin index, and so its consumption results in a lower insulin release. For that reason, and because of its higher fiber and micronutrient content, whole-wheat bread is claimed to be healthier than white bread.

What the media frequently fails to mention is that the actual differences between white bread and whole-wheat bread are relatively small. Yes, whole-wheat bread has a higher fiber content — but this content pales compared to that of many fruits and vegetables. You most definitely do not have to eat whole-wheat products to get enough fiber in your diet! And yes, white bread does lose more micronutrients during processing — but those micronutrients are often reintroduced later (the bread is then called "enriched").

The Truth: While some people are sensitive to wheat, the gluten content isn't necessarily to blame, and other foods may also be implicated. Bread, nor any other food, will inherently cause weight gain unless its consumption puts you in a caloric surplus. Though whole-wheat bread is claimed to be far healthier than white bread, they are not that different, and neither contains high levels of fiber or micronutrients.

Myth #12 HFCS is far worse than sugar

High fructose corn syrup (HFCS) is a blend of both glucose and fructose commonly used to sweeten food products.

Early evidence led to the belief that fructose could cause fatty-liver disease, as well as insulin resistance and obesity. By extension, HFCS is frequently said to be unhealthy, since it is high in fructose.

The reality is that there isn't always more fructose in HFCS than in sugar. Liquid HFCS has a fructose content of 42–55%. Sucrose, also known as table sugar, is 50% fructose. The difference (-8% to +5%) is too slight to matter.

The Truth: HFCS and table sugar are remarkably similar from a health perspective. Though HFCS may sometimes contain more fructose, the difference is negligible.

Myth #13 Fresh is more nutritious than frozen

Fresh produce has a natural appeal to many people. It just *sounds* better than "canned" or "frozen" fruits and vegetables. But just because a food is "fresh" does not necessarily mean it's more nutritious.

Fresh produce is defined as anything that is "postharvest ripened" (if it ripens during transport) or "vine-ripened" (if it is picked and sold ripe: at a farmer's fresh market or at a farmer's roadside fruit stand, for instance).

Frozen produce is generally vine-ripened before undergoing minimal processing prior to freezing. Most vegetables and some fruits undergo blanching in hot water for a few minutes before freezing, in order to inactivate enzymes that may cause unfavorable changes in color, smell, flavor, and nutritional value.

While there are some differences between fresh and frozen for *select* nutrients in *select* fruits and veggies, overall, they have very similar nutritional content.

The Truth: While there can be some nutrient differences between fresh and frozen produce, the overall differences are small. Pick whichever suits your taste, budget, and lifestyle.

Myth #14 Food nutrients are always superior to supplemental nutrients

How often have you heard the claim that natural, whole foods are always better than synthetic supplements? In general, the word "natural" has a positive connotation whereas "synthetic" or "chemical" has a negative one.

The truth, of course, is not so clear-cut. Some compounds are more effective in supplemental form. One example is the curcumin in turmeric. On its own, your body cannot absorb it well; but taken in liposomal form or supplemented with piperine, a black pepper extract, curcumin sees its bioavailability increase dramatically.

The same goes for vitamins. For instance, phylloquinone (K_1) is tightly bound to membranes in plants and so is more bioavailable in supplemental form. Likewise, folic acid (supplemental B_9) is more bioavailable than folate (B_9 naturally present in foods), though that may not always be a good thing.

The Truth: With regard notably to vitamins, foods are not always superior to supplements.

Myth #15 You should eat "clean"

This statement is not so much a myth as a jumble of misconceptions. First, people seldom agree on what "clean" actually means. For some, it means shunning specific foods for religious or ethical reasons. For others, it means avoiding highly processed foods. For others still, it means eating organic. One common point of clean diets is their focus on exclusion: they tell you what clean eating is by telling you what *not* to eat.

Veganism can be considered a prototypal clean diet, as it shuns all animal products both for ethical reasons and for better health. But although vegans and vegetarians do tend to be healthier on average, this may be due to reasons unrelated to food. For instance, people who stick to a vegetarian diet are more likely to also stick to an exercise regimen and neither drink in excess nor smoke.

As it stands, compared to people eating a varied omnivorous diet, vegans (and, to a lesser extent, vegetarians) are more likely to get less than the optimal amount of some nutrients, such as L-carnitine or vitamin B. However, those nutrients can easily be supplemented — nowadays, there are even plant-based options for EPA, DHA, and vitamin D_3.

But animal products are not the only "unclean" foods for clean-diet proselytizers. You cannot simply "eat your veggies" — you need to make sure they are organic. This is presented as self-evident, on the principle that "natural" is good whereas "synthetic" is bad. So far, however, what few studies have investigated the effect of organic food on clinical health outcomes have failed to consistently link organic foods, plants, or animal, to better health.

To be more precise, most observational studies have found no association between eating organic and a decrease in risk of eczema, wheezing, atopic sensitization, or overall incidence of cancer. One observational study reported that eating mostly organic food might decrease the risk of developing non-Hodgkin lymphoma in women. Another reported that, compared to non-organic dairy products, organic dairy products might lower the risk of eczema in young children.

None of this proves that a link cannot exist between organic food and better health, but the organic-versus-conventional debate is complex and can change both with the foods under scrutiny and with the individuals eating them.

One misconception is that no synthetic substance can be used to grow organic crops, whereas the National List of Allowed and Prohibited Substances makes some exceptions. Another misconception is that no pesticide can be used to grow organic crops, whereas natural pesticides exist, are used to grow organic crops, and are not always better for the consumer or the environment.

Pesticide residues in food are a valid concern, though it should be noted that the Pesticide Data Program (PDP) of the United States Department of Agriculture (USDA) has consistently found that the vast majority of the food on the market contain either no detectable residues or residues below the tolerable limits set by the Environmental Protection Agency (EPA).

While the USDA does not currently test for residues of pesticides commonly use on organic foods, it does test for residues of pesticides *not* approved and some approved for *limited* application. Unsurprisingly, pesticide residues were most often found in non-organic foods, but when found, pesticide residues were similarly low in both organic and non-organic foods.

To add another wrinkle, there is some evidence that even very low doses of pesticides might still elicit physiological effects. These effects, be they beneficial, neutral, or harmful, and be they from organic or conventional pesticides, are not well studied. So, what is a consumer to do? The practical solution is quite simple: rinsing, peeling when possible, and cooking can reduce the amount of pesticide left on your produce, whether this produce is organic or not.

Is our food clean enough yet? Not quite. Some "clean eating" gurus recommend that you only eat your food raw, so as not to "denature" its nutrients. As an absolute, this rule is a myth. Raw milk can contain harmful bacteria. Raw eggs contain avidin, a protein that can bind biotin and thus lead to biotin deficiency if consumed frequently. Cooking can reduce the nitrate content of vegetables (bad) but also their oxalate content (good). You cannot generalize.

It's easy to see how one can push the "clean eating" obsession too far, even all the way into orthorexia nervosa, a disorder in which you become obsessed with eating healthy.[65] It doesn't mean that all foods are equal, and you certainly should favor whole foods over highly processed foods — most of which are nutrient-poor, calorie-dense, and easy to overeat — but you shouldn't fear that eating anything but raw organic veggies is going to drastically shorten your lifespan (whereas too much stress can.

The Truth: "Clean eating" is tough to define, as gurus do not even agree on which foods are clean and which are not. Stick to the basics. Favor whole foods (but don't feel like any small amount of processed foods will kill you), eat organic if you wish to and can afford it, peel or wash all your vegetables and fruits, and avoid stressing too much about what you eat, since stress *can* shorten your lifespan.

Myth #16 You should "detox" regularly

"Detox diets" are the ultimate manifestation of the "clean eating" obsession. Such diets commonly limit foods to plant-based juices, sometimes seasoned with a supplement. After a few days of that regimen, you are supposed to be cleansed of …

Well, those detox diet companies do not really know. A 2009 investigation of ten companies found they couldn't name a single "toxin" eliminated by any of their fifteen products — let alone prove that their products worked. Strictly speaking, toxins are plant- or animal-based substances poisonous to humans; but for many detox gurus, "toxins" also include heavy metals … and everything synthetic: not just toxicants (man-made poisons, such as pollutants or pesticides), but also preservatives, high-fructose corn syrup, etc.

Alas, even when a substance really *is* noxious, a "detox diet" will not help. Acute toxicity would likely constitute a medical emergency, whereas chronic toxicity can be handled better by a well-fed body — not one weakened by a severely hypocaloric diet. The liver, kidneys, lungs, and other organs work around the clock to remove harmful substances and excrete the waste products of metabolism. By reducing your intake of the nutrients, they need to perform these functions, a detox diet can hinder your body's natural detoxification process! If you wish to promote this process, your best bet is to load up with various foods that can help these organs work optimally, such as cruciferous and other fibrous veggies.

Detox diets are not necessarily safe, either. Every now and then a case report emerges about potential risks, such as kidney damage from green smoothies or liver failure from detox teas.

But if "detox diets" are more likely to harm than help, what explains their current popularity? One answer is: quick weight loss. Deprive your body from carbohydrate and you can exhaust its glycogen stores in as little as 24 hours. The resulting loss of several pounds can convince you the diet had a positive effect. When the diet ends and you resume your regular eating habits, however, the glycogen and associated water come rushing back in, and with them the pounds you'd shed.

The Truth: Focus on sustainable health habits, such as eating nutritious food daily. Ample protein, leafy greens, and foods chock-full of vitamins and minerals are not just tastier than anything a "detox diet" has to offer, they are also way better for you (and your liver detoxification pathways, ironically). A detox diet might make you feel better, but that is usually because of the increased vegetable and fruit intake, not because any form of detoxification is taking place.

Myth #17 Eat more often to boost your metabolism

It is easy to trace this myth back to its origin. Digestion does raise your metabolism a little, so many people believe that eating less food more often keeps your metabolism elevated.

But evidence shows that, given an equal amount of daily calories, the number of meals largely makes no difference in fat loss. Moreover, some studies suggest that having smaller meals more often makes it harder to feel full, potentially leading to increased food intake. Your metabolism can fluctuate based on the size of the meal, so fewer but larger meals means a larger spike in metabolism. Over the course of a day or week, given an equal number of calories, the number of meals doesn't seem to matter — it all evens out.

The Truth: Digestion does slightly increase your metabolic rate, but meal frequency has less effect than the total caloric content of the food consumed.

Myth #18 You need to eat breakfast

"Breakfast is the most important meal of the day" is something we have all heard before from parents, health bloggers, doctors, and ad campaigns. But the health advantages of consuming a regular breakfast has been overhyped.

People who are #TeamBreakfast have pointed to observational studies showing a higher BMI in breakfast skippers. However, clinical trials have pointed to personal preference being a critical factor. Some people will subconsciously compensate for all the calories they skipped at breakfast, while others will not feel cravings of the same magnitude. In one trial, women who did not habitually eat breakfast were made to consume it; they gained nearly 2 pounds over a 4-week period. Individual responses do vary, so do not try to force yourself into an eating pattern that does not sit well with you or that you can't sustain — it may end up backfiring.

Another popular claim is that skipping breakfast can crash your metabolism. But studies in both lean and overweight individuals have shown that skipping breakfast does not *inherently* slow your *resting metabolic rate* (RMR).

One area where the "don't skip breakfast" mantra might hold true is in people with impaired glucose regulation. These individuals might benefit from consuming breakfast to achieve better day-to-day glucose management."

The Truth: You don't *need* to eat breakfast to be healthy or lose weight. You should base your breakfast consumption on your preferences and personal goals. Feel free to experiment to see if you want to make skipping breakfast a habit.

Myth #19 To lose fat, do not eat before bed

Some studies show a fat-loss advantage in early eaters, others in late eaters. Overall, early eaters seem to have a *slight* advantage — nothing impressive. Trials, however, imperfectly reflect real life. In real life, there are two main reasons why eating at night might hinder fat loss, and both are linked to an increase in your daily caloric intake.

The first reason is the simplest: if, instead of going directly to bed, we first indulge in a snack, then the calories from that snack are calories we might have done without.

The second reason is that, when we get tired, we tend to eat to keep going, with a predilection for snack foods or tasty treats. So, if we stay awake at night — specially to work or study, but even just to watch TV — we are more likely to eat, not out of hunger, but to help fight sleepiness.

The Truth: Eating *late* will not make you gain fat unless it drives you to eat *more*. It can also be harder to resist tasty, high-calorie snacks after a long day.

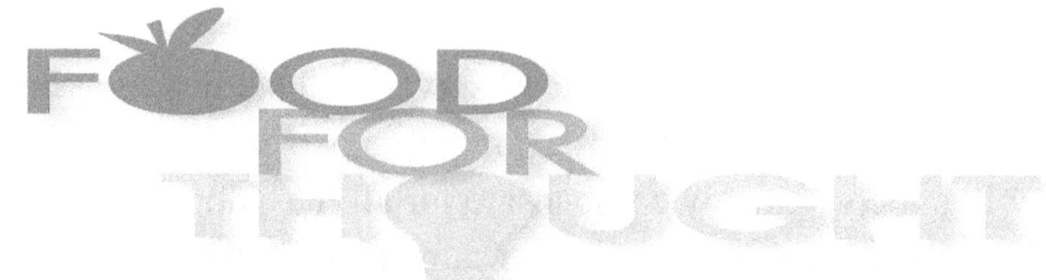

WORKSHEETS

Simple Meal Creator

PROTEIN	VEGGIES	STARCH	FAT	FLAVOR

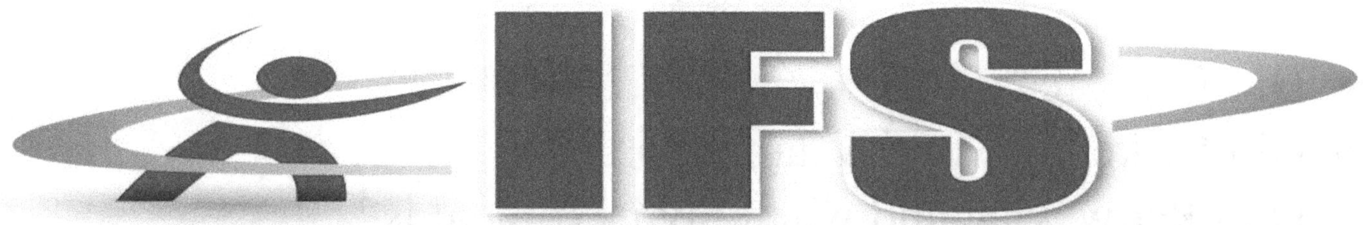

Awesome IFS friendly meal

Why is this meal so good?

- ❏ Lean protein
- ❏ Colorful fruits and/or vegetables
- ❏ Healthy fats
- ❏ Makes you feel great
- ❏ Something else:

____

What needs to happen?

What do i need to do or prepare it?

- ❏ Prep in advance
- ❏ Have food on hand
- ❏ Go shopping
- ❏ Something else:

____

Expanding on success

How could I do more of this?

- ❏ Cook in bulk
- ❏ Get some Tupperware
- ❏ Get a health meal delivery service
- ❏ Try new recipes
- ❏ Something else:

____

Your List of Daily Questions/Reflections:

- Did I eat breakfast?
- Did I take my Multi Vitamin?
- Do I know what and when my next meal is?
- Did I journal my food intake and/or thoughts?
- Did I find ways to add in 'Surprise Exercise' every hour?
- Did I remain Positive and/or Realistic?
- Did I plan for meals and challenging situations?
- Did I find 10- minutes to be with my thoughts?
- Did I monitor my self-talk?
- Was I able to respond to situations, rather than react?
- How many times did I eat today?
- Did I eat balanced meals (P,C,F)?
- Did I eat every 3-4 hours (no more than 5 hours between meals)?
- Did I consume quality calories today?
- Did I limit "junk" food today?
- How much time did I spend reading today?
- What were my reasons to smile today?
- When was I the most alert and energetic?
- How did my energy affect what I ate?
- How did what I ate affect my energy?
- How did my thinking affect my energy?
- How did my thinking affect my food choices?
- How did I respond to challenges and setbacks?
- What will I do next to move forward?

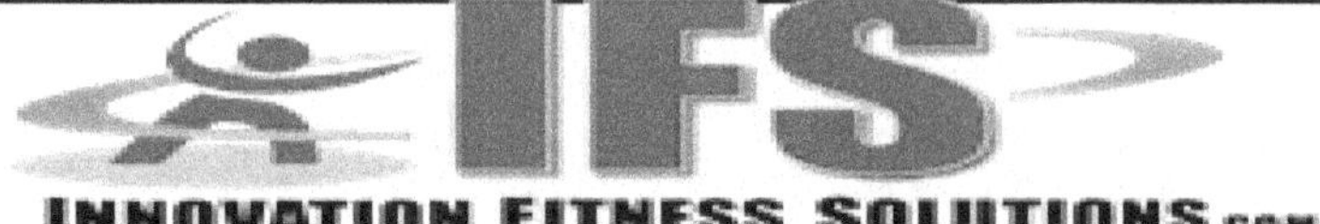

I. Short Range Goal: _______________________________________

    A. Step 1: _______________________________________

    B. Step 2: _______________________________________

    C. Step 3: _______________________________________

II. Short Range Goal: _______________________________________

    A. Step 1: _______________________________________

    B. Step 2: _______________________________________

    C. Step 3: _______________________________________

III. Short Range Goal: _______________________________________

    A. Step 1: _______________________________________

    B. Step 2: _______________________________________

    C. Step 3: _______________________________________

IV. Short Range Goal: _______________________________________

    A. Step 1: _______________________________________

    B. Step 2: _______________________________________

    C. Step 3: _______________________________________

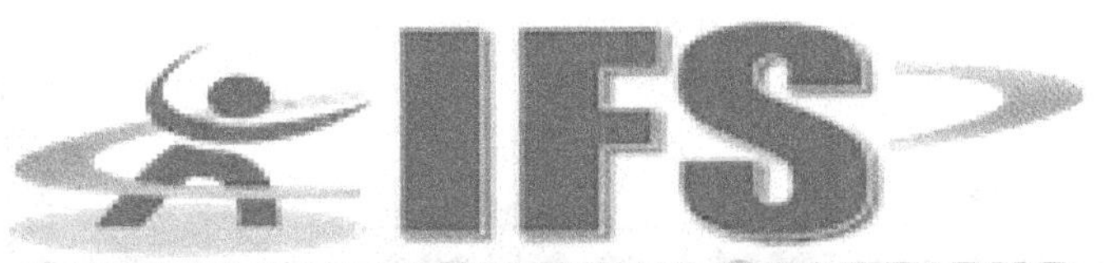

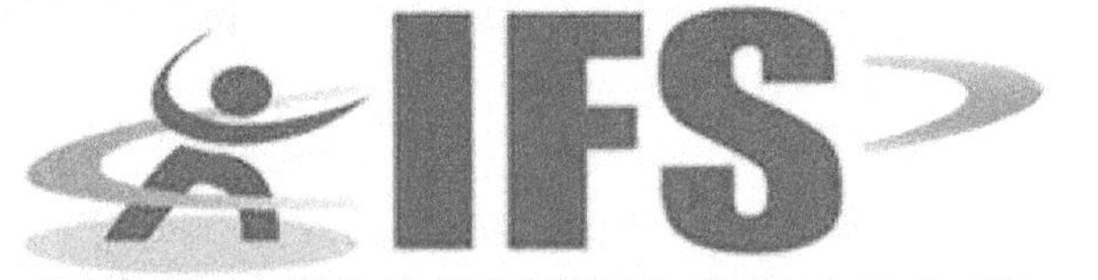

Weight	Waist	Strength	Interpretation	Recommendation
Decreasing	Decreasing	Increasing	Fat loss is occurring. Perfect spot.	Stay the course.
Decreasing	Decreasing	Decreasing	Fat loss is occurring.	Stay the course or consider decreasing deficit.
Decreasing	Decreasing	Same	Fat loss is occurring.	Stay the course.
Decreasing	Increasing	Increasing	Fat loss is likely occurring. Measurements may have been off or increases in lean mass around the waist are occurring.	Stay the course.
Decreasing	Increasing	Decreasing	Fat loss may be occurring, but hard to interpret.	If nothing has changed from previous training/nutrition, then stay the course.
Decreasing	Increasing	Same	Fat loss is likely occurring.	Stay the course.
Increasing	Decreasing	Increasing	Fat loss is either occurring very slowly or the trainee is getting accustomed to a new carbohydrate intake.	Consider increasing caloric deficit, unless this was an intentional increase in carbohydrates. In that case, weight will level off and then reverse.
Increasing	Decreasing	Decreasing	Hard to interpret. Could be either measurements, but likely losing strength and gaining fat.	Check again in a week.
Increasing	Decreasing	Same	Hard to interpret. Could be erratic measurements.	Use best judgment, but would likely decrease calories with a more aggressive deficit to ensure fat loss is occurring.
Increasing	Increasing	Increasing	Fat/muscle gain. You are likely in a caloric surplus.	Increase caloric deficit or switch focus to muscle gain
Increasing	Increasing	Decreasing	Fat gain is occurring.	Lower calories and look into training routine.
Increasing	Increasing	Same	Fat gain is occurring.	Lower calories and look into training routine.
Same	Decreasing	Increasing	Simultaneous fat loss/muscle gain.	Consider increasing deficit to increase fat loss. Good place to settle at for clients relatively close to weight goal but who cannot decrease calories further.
Same	Decreasing	Decreasing	Fat loss with weight lagging behind. Either there is "bloat" occurring or scale will catch up.	Stay the course for a week or two. If you feel "bloated" during this time, you're likely going to see an increase in the scale number.
Same	Decreasing	Same	Fat loss with weight lagging behind. Either there is "bloat" occurring or scale will catch up.	Stay the course. Check back in a week or two. Weight will likely drop or strength will likely increase.
Same	Increasing	Decreasing	Simultaneous fat gain/muscle loss. Usually occurs during a break, e.g. when on a caloric surplus with little training.	Increase caloric deficit and examine training.
Same	Increasing	Increasing	Simultaneous fat loss/muscle gain. Either previous reading may have been wrong or scale will eventually catch up.	Use best judgment. Increase caloric deficit if fat loss has seemed slow lately.
Same	Increasing	Same	Simultaneous fat gain/muscle loss. Usually occurs during a break. e.g. when on a caloric surplus with little training.	Increase caloric deficit.

HABIT1	DRINK	Drink two glasses of water upon waking. Add at least 32 additional ounces to your current total throughout the day.
HABIT2	PLAN	Plan your meals for the week, either on Sunday or Monday. Grid your free meals ahead of time.
HABIT3	SHOP	Go shopping for the food on your plan, either on Sunday or Monday.
HABIT4	COOK	Prepare, cook, and portion the food on your plan on Sunday or Monday.
HABIT5	JOURNAL	Keep a daily food journal. Review your food journal weekly, either on Sunday or Monday.
HABIT6	PROTEIN	Make sure you're getting protein at every meal. Shoot for three-quarters of a gram of protein per pound of target bodyweight, per day.
HABIT7	CALORIES	Review your food journal for total calories consumed. Compare your total calories to your weekly weight change.
HABIT8	SLOW	Eat slowly. A meal should take at least 15 minutes.
HABIT9	80%	Stop eating when you're 80% full.
HABIT10	HEALTHY FAT	Make sure you're getting good fats at most meals. Add good fat to meals you normally feel hungry after and see if that helps you feel full.
HABIT11	QUALITY CARBS	Check the quality of your carbohydrates. Are you getting most of your carbohydrates from brown rice, quinoa, brown rice pasta, sprouted-grain bread, fruit, and vegetables?
HABIT12	GRATITUDE	Keep a gratitude journal - every day, write down one thing you like about your body, are proud of about your body, or are grateful for about your body.

SIGNS YOUR NUTRITION PLAN IS WORKING

The scale and your body weight don't always give you the full picture of progress.

Here are some better ways to tell that your nutrition plan is working.

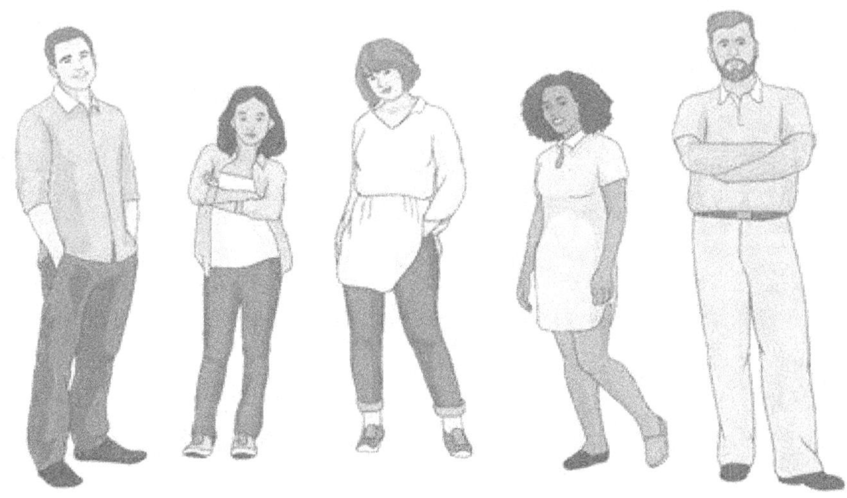

☐ You're satisfied after meals   ☐ You're in a better mood   ☐ You're sleeping better

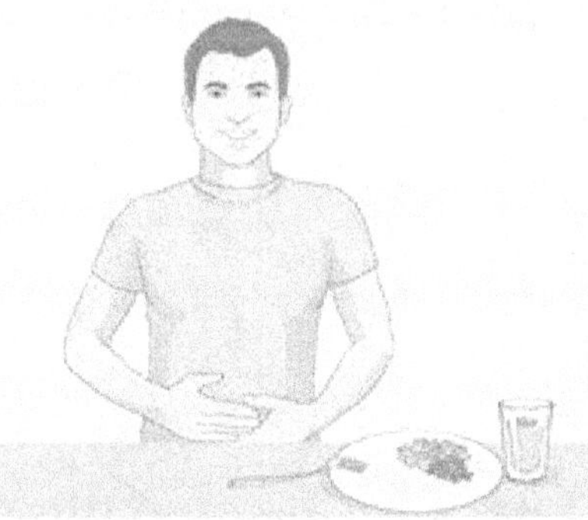
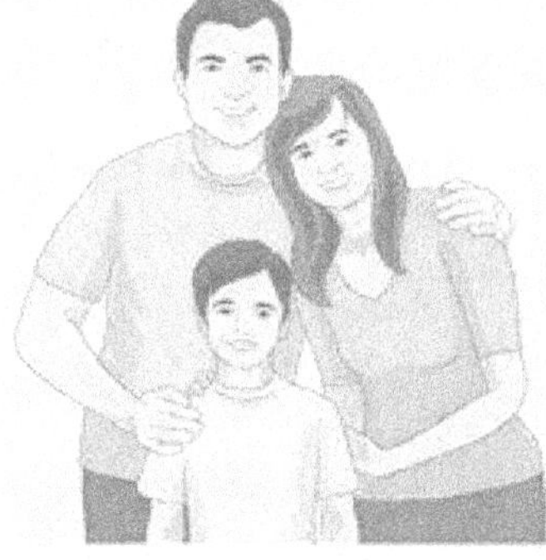
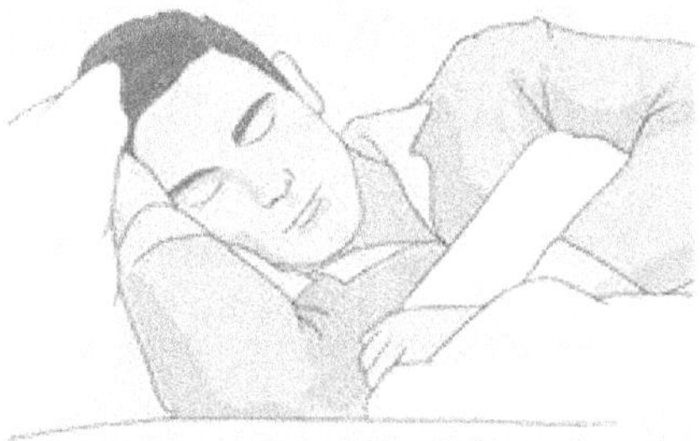

☐ You have more energy, more consistently   ☐ You're stronger and have more endurance   ☐ Your habits feel more like a lifestyle than a "diet"

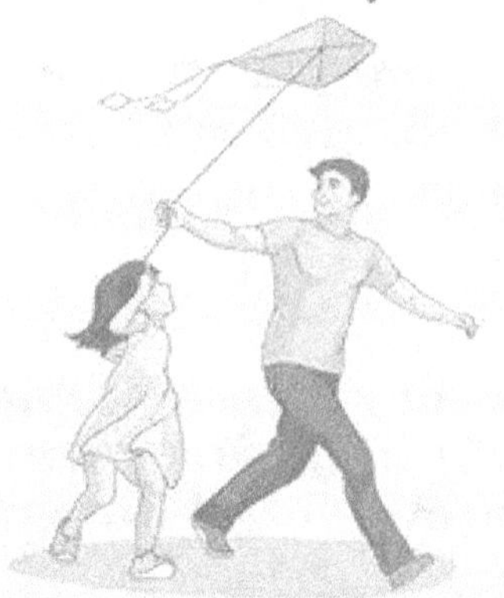
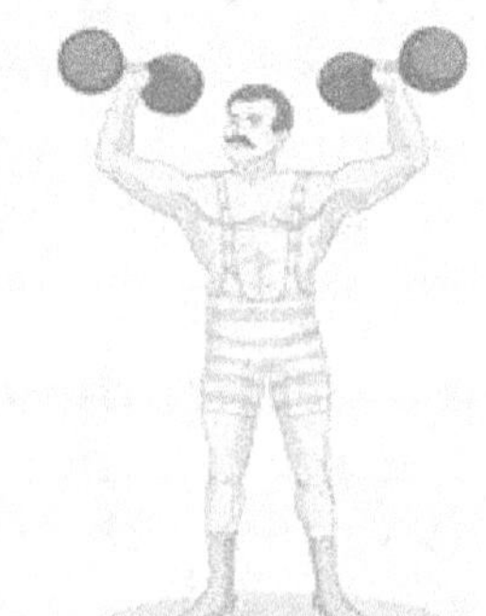
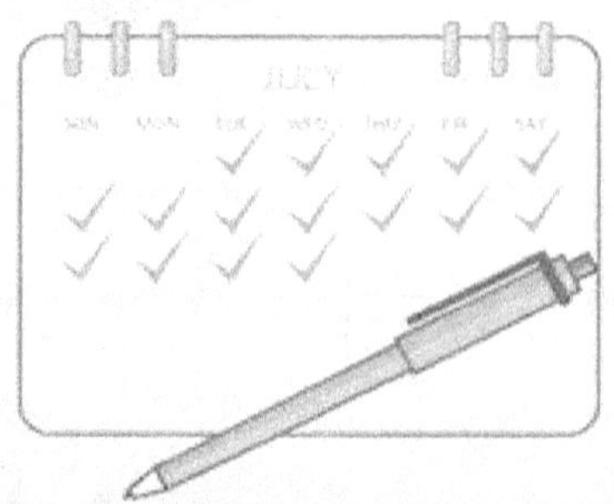

PHYSICAL

- ☐ You have less pain -- maybe you're even pain-free!
- ☐ You have less inflammation (e.g. joint stiffness, autoimmune fare-ups, etc.).
- ☐ You have better mobility (e.g. a better range of motion on a certain exercise, or feeling more mobile in general).
- ☐ You take fewer medications, or a lower dose of them.
- ☐ You have better blood work or other lab tests.
- ☐ You have fewer digestive problems.
- ☐ You heal and recover from injury or illness more quickly.

PERFORMANCE

- ☐ You perform better athletically.
- ☐ You can do daily-life tasks better (e.g. lifting things into the car, carrying groceries, managing a dog pulling on a leash, etc.).

EMOTIONAL / MENTAL

- ☐ You feel more confident.
- ☐ You feel like change is possible.
- ☐ You feel better about your choices.
- ☐ You feel more knowledgeable.
- ☐ You feel clearer about your goals and the path to get to them.
- ☐ You feel mentally more "on" -- you're thinking more clearly, with less fuzziness or forgetfulness.
- ☐ You feel more open to trying new things.
- ☐ You feel happier and more positive.
- ☐ You feel motivated (e.g. motivated to train, motivated to persist)!

APPEARANCE

- ☐ Your skin looks better (e.g. less acne; fewer rashes; general improvement).
- ☐ Your hair and fingernails are stronger.
- ☐ You look generally "fitter" / more athletic.
- ☐ You're walking taller and more confidently.

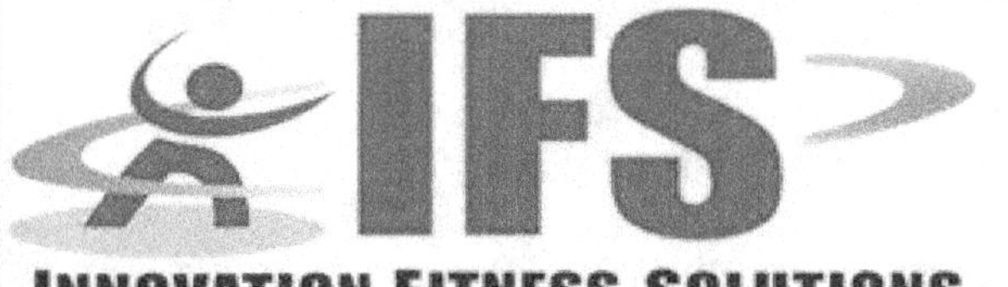

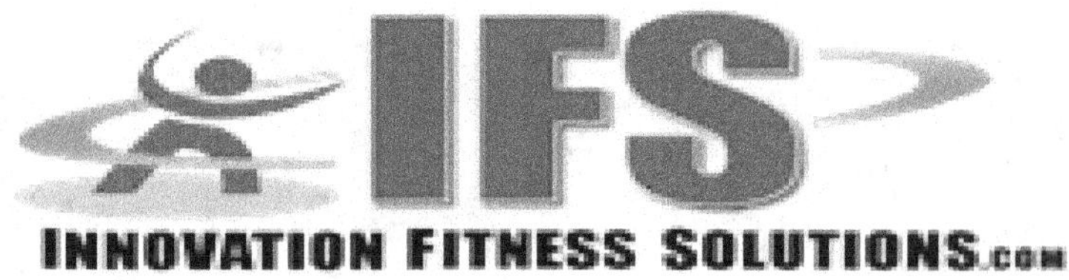

Focus –

1. How much time do I spend reading per day?

2. How do I speak to myself during stressful times (actual phrases)?

3. What do I wish I could tell myself during stressful, busy times?

4. What is my current self-care ritual?

5. What is my best food habit? Worst?

6. What do I honestly believe that I deserve?

7. How often do I think about the repercussions of my self-talk on my happiness?

Food –

1. How many feedings have I been having per day?

2. What is a typical weeks' food intake list?

Healthy / Low Calorie	Healthy / High Calorie
Unhealthy / Low Calorie	Unhealthy / High Calorie

3. How does my "Weekday Me" differ from my "Weekend Me"?

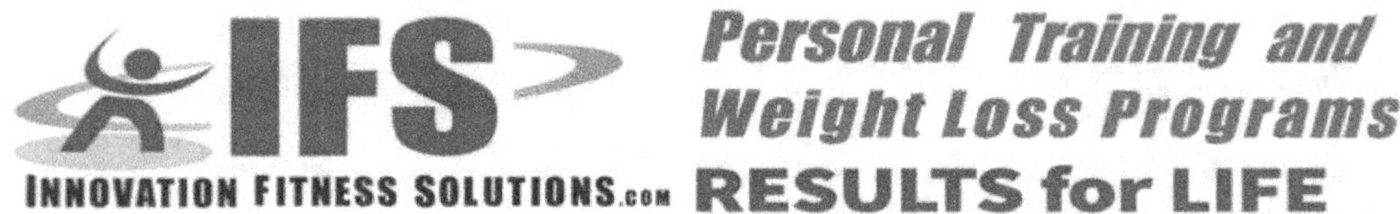

4. What % of my meals do I prepare and eat at home?

5. How many grams of Protein and Fiber do I eat per day? Water in oz?

6. How often do I shop for food and plan my meals?

7. How often do I consider the repercussions of my food choices as they relate to health, performance and body composition change?

Fitness –

1. What is my best fitness habit? Worst?

2. How many strength workouts do I perform per week?

3. How many steps (amount of activity) do I perform daily?

4. What level of focus and intensity do I bring to my training?

5. How would I rate my exercise form?

6. How much time do I spend sitting or laying down?

7. How many hours do I sleep per night? Do I feel rested?

8. Do I have any recurring injuries or tweaks?

9. How often do I consider my movement levels as they relate to my pain levels and performance output?

Who do I need to become to get what I want?

The 4 questions for change

What are the **advantages of** changing?

What are the **disadvantages of changing?**

What are the **advantages of NOT** changing?

What are the **disadvantages of NOT** changing?

The 4 methods of change

START a completely new action

STOP doing something entirely

Do **MORE** of something

Do **LESS** of something

The 3 questions for Action

What Actions **can I** take?

What **can I** read?

Who **can I** ask?

The 3 Lies we tell ourselves

I can't do this

I am alone

It will always be this way

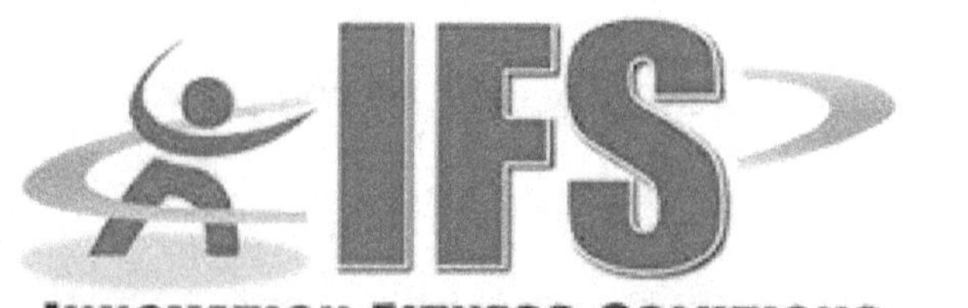

IFS Meal Plan Template

Starch Choices

15 g CHO, 3 g PRO, 1 g Fat and 80 Calories

Starch	Serving Size
Beans	½ cup cooked
Bread Products	1 oz
Cereal	½ cup cooked
Grains	½ cup cooked
Pasta	1/3 cup cooked
Potatoes	½ cup cooked
Rice	1/3 cup cooked
Snack foods	¾ to 1 oz

Non-starchy Vegetable Choices

5 g CHO, 2 g PRO, 0 g Fat and 25 Calories

Vegetable	Serving Size
Cooked Vegetables	½ cup
Raw Vegetables	1 cup
Vegetable Juice	½ cup

Fruit Choices

15 g CHO, 0 g PRO, 0 g Fat and 60 Calories

Fruit	Serving Size
Canned or Frozen Fruit	½ cup
Dried Fruit	2 Tbsp
Fresh Fruit	¾ to 1 cup
Unsweetened Fruit Juice	½ cup

Lean Protein Choices

0 g CHO, 7 g PRO, 2 g Fat and 45 Calories

Protein	Serving Size
Chicken Without Skin	1 oz
Cottage Cheese	1 oz
Egg Whites	1
Fish (salmon, tuna)	1 oz
Ground Beef (90% Lean)	1 oz
Lamb	1 oz
Turkey Without Skin	1 oz
Veal	1 oz

Medium-Fat Choices

0 g CHO, 7 g PRO, 5 g Fat and 75 Calories

Protein	Serving Size
Chicken with Skin	1 oz
Egg	1
Feta Cheese	1 oz
Fish (fried)	1 oz
Ground Beef (85% lean)	1 oz
Mozzarella Cheese	1 oz

High-Fat Choices

0 g CHO, 7 g PRO, 8 g Fat and 100 Calories

Protein	Serving Size
American Cheese	1 oz
Bacon	1 oz
Cheddar Cheese	1 oz
Parmesan	1 oz
Processed Sandwich Meats	1 oz

<table>
<tr><td colspan="2">Fat Choices</td></tr>
</table>

5 g Fat and 45 Calories

Fat	Serving Size
Almond Milk	1 cup
Avocado	2 Tbsp
Bacon	1 slice
Butter	1 Tbsp
Cream	2 Tbsp
Cream Cheese	1 ½ Tbsp
Coconut Oil	1 tsp
Margarine	1 Tbsp
Mayonnaise	1 Tbsp
Nuts	6-12
Nut Butters	1 ½ tsp
Oils	1 tsp
Salad Dressing	2 Tbsp
Seeds	1 ½ Tbsp

<table>
<tr><td colspan="2">Dairy Choices</td></tr>
</table>

Dairy	Calories
8 oz of Skim or 1%	0-3 g fat and 100 calories
8 oz 2%	5 g fat and 120 calories
8 oz whole milk	8 g fat and 160 calories

1500 Calorie Sample Menu					
Food	**Serving Size**	**CHO (g)**	**PRO (g)**	**Fat (g)**	**Calories**
dotfit LeanMR	2 scoops	24	21	2	180
Skim Milk	8 oz	0	0	3	100
Oatmeal	1 cup cooked	30	6	2	160
Fresh Blueberries	¾ cup	15	0	0	60
Chicken (no skin)	3 oz	0	21	6	135
Broccoli	1 cup cooked	10	4	0	50
Brown Rice	1/3 cup cooked	15	3	1	80
Olive Oil	1 tsp	0	0	5	45
Plain Greek Yogurt	6 oz	0	0	3	100
Raw veggies	1 ½ cup	10	4	0	50
Turkey (no skin)	3 oz	0	21	6	135
Tomatoes & Peppers	1 ½ cup cooked	15	6	0	75
Whole Wheat Pasta	1/3 cup cooked	15	3	1	80
Rice Cakes	2	30	6	3	160
Peanut Butter	1 Tbsp	0	0	10	90
Totals		**164**	**95**	**42**	**1500**

Food	Serving Size	CHO (g)	PRO (g)	Fat (g)	Calories
dotfit LeanMR	2 scoops	24	21	2	180
2% Milk	8 oz	0	0	5	120
Mixed Berries	1 cup	15	0	0	60
Almond Butter	1 Tbsp	0	0	10	90
Chia Seeds	1 Tbsp	0	0	10	90
Chicken (no skin)	4 oz	0	28	8	180
Broccoli	1 cup cooked	10	4	0	50
Brown Rice	2/3 cup cooked	30	6	2	160
Olive Oil	1 Tbsp	0	0	15	135
Yogurt	6 oz	0	0	3	100
Cottage Cheese	2 oz	0	14	4	90
Chicken (no skin)	4 oz	0	28	8	180
Mozzarella Cheese	1 oz	0	7	5	75
Spinach & Tomato	1 ½ cup cooked	15	6	2	160
Whole Wheat Bread	2 slices	30	6	2	160
Oatmeal	1 cup cooked	30	6	2	160
Grapes	1 cup	15	0	0	60
Peanut Butter	1 ½ tsp	0	0	5	45
Totals		**169**	**126**	**81**	**2010**

Food	Serving Size	CHO (g)	PRO (g)	Fat (g)	Calories
dotfit LeanMR	2 scoops	24	21	2	180
2% Milk	8 oz	0	0	5	120
Eggs	3	0	21	15	225
Chia Seeds	1 Tbsp	0	0	10	90
Chicken (no skin)	5 oz	0	32	10	225
Asparagus & Broccoli	2 cups cooked	20	8	0	100
Quinoa	1 cup	45	9	3	240
Banana	1 Medium	15	0	0	60
Peanut Butter	1 Tbsp	0	0	10	90
Ground Beef	4 oz	0	28	8	180
Shredded Parmesan	2 oz	0	14	16	200
Whole Wheat Pasta	1 cup cooked	45	9	3	240
Salad w/ veggies	1 cup raw	10	4	0	50
Dressing	2 Tbsp	0	0	5	45
Mixed Vegetables	1 cup raw	5	2	0	25
Hummus	1 ½ Tbsp	0	0	15	135
Totals		**194**	**154**	**119**	**2500**

Food	Serving Size	CHO (g)	PRO (g)	Fat (g)	Calories
dotfit LeanMR	2 scoops	24	21	2	180
2% Milk	8 oz	0	0	5	120
Starbucks w/ Creamer	16 oz	24	2	2	120
Blueberry Muffin	1	55	6	12	350
Fried/Breaded Chicken	4 oz	10	32	20	300
Baked Potato	1 Whole	30	4	2	160
Butter	2 Tbsp	0	0	10	90
Side Salad	1 ½ cup raw	15	9	0	75
Dressing	2 Tbsp	0	0	5	45
Iced Tea	12 oz	32	0	0	100
Almonds	½ cup	0	0	15	135
Pepperoni Pizza	2 Slices	68	20	24	596
Coke	8 oz	26	0	0	80
Meal Replacement Bar	1	15	15	5	160
Totals		**289**	**109**	**97**	**2511**

Food	Serving Size	CHO (g)	PRO (g)	Fat (g)	Calories
dotfit LeanMR	2 scoops	24	21	2	180
2% Milk	8 oz	0	0	5	120
Mixed Berries	2 cups	30	0	0	120
Almond Butter	2 Tbsp	0	0	20	180
Chia Seeds	1 Tbsp	0	0	10	90
Chicken (no skin)	5 oz	0	32	10	225
Spinach	1 cup raw	5	2	0	25
Chickpeas	¼ cup	15	10	4	125
Mixed Veggies	1 cup raw	5	2	0	25
Oil & Vinegar	1 Tbsp	0	0	5	90
Dried Cranberries	1 Tbsp	15	0	0	60
Almonds	¼ cup	0	0	15	135
Yogurt	6 oz	0	0	3	100
Meal Replacement Bar	1	15	15	5	160
Granola	¼ cup	15	3	1	80
Chicken (no skin)	5 oz	0	32	10	225
Brown Rice	2 cup cooked	90	18	6	480
Stir Fry Veggies	1 cup cooked	10	4	0	50
Olive Oil	1 Tbsp	0	0	10	90
Banana	1 medium	15	0	0	60
Peanut Butter	2 Tbsp	0	0	20	180
Air Popped Popcorn	1 cup cooked	15	3	1	80
Totals		**279**	**144**	**134**	**3015**

3000 Calorie Sample Menu – Typical Day					
Food	**Serving Size**	**CHO (g)**	**PRO (g)**	**Fat (g)**	**Calories**
dotfit LeanMR	2 scoops	24	21	2	180
2% Milk	8 oz	0	0	5	120
Starbucks w/ Creamer	16 oz	24	2	2	120
Bagel	1	60	6	3	220
Cream Cheese	2 Tbsp	0	0	15	180
Eggs	3	0	21	6	225
Fried/Breaded Chicken	4 oz	10	32	20	300
Baked Potato	1 Whole	30	4	2	160
Butter	2 Tbsp	0	0	10	90
Side Salad	2 cup raw	20	12	0	100
Dressing	2 Tbsp	0	0	5	45
Iced Tea	12 oz	32	0	0	100
Almonds	½ cup	0	0	15	135
Meal Replacement Bar	1	15	15	5	160
Pepperoni Pizza	2 Slices	68	20	24	596
Coke	8 oz	26	0	0	80
Yogurt	6 oz	0	0	3	100
Granola	¼ cup	15	3	1	80
Chips	1 bag	30	4	2	160
Totals		**354**	**140**	**120**	**3151**

 Innovation Fitness Solutions – Achievers Success Guide

ENERGY BALANCE

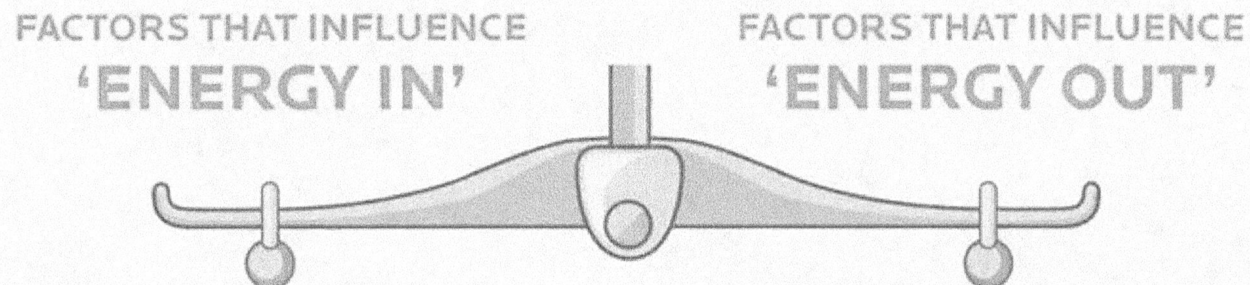

FACTORS THAT INFLUENCE **'ENERGY IN'**	FACTORS THAT INFLUENCE **'ENERGY OUT'**
APPETITE Influenced by hormones that regulate appetite and satiety	**ENERGY BURNED AT REST** Influenced by body size, hormonal status, dieting history, genetic factors, health status, sleep quality, age
FOOD CONSUMED Influenced by availability, palatability, energy density, sleep quality, education, socioeconomic status, culture	**ENERGY BURNED THROUGH EXERCISE** Influenced by exercise ability, intensity, duration, frequency, type, environment, as well as hormonal status and sleep quality
CALORIES ABSORBED Influenced by macronutrient intake, food prep, age, personal microbiome, health status, energy status	**ENERGY BURNED BY NON-EXERCISE ACTIVITY** Influenced by health status, energy status, stress levels, hormonal status, occupation, leisure activities, genetic factors
PSYCHOLOGICAL FACTORS Influenced by stress levels, mindset, perceived control, self-esteem, sleep quality	**ENERGY BURNED METABOLIZING FOOD** Influenced by macronutrient makeup and how processed the food is

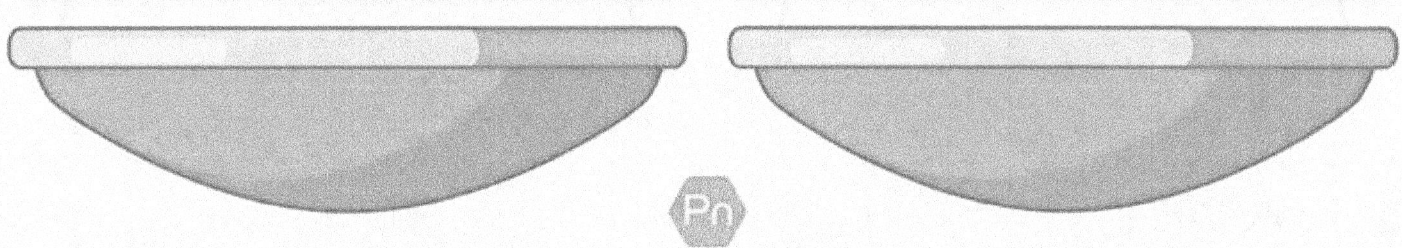

January 2021